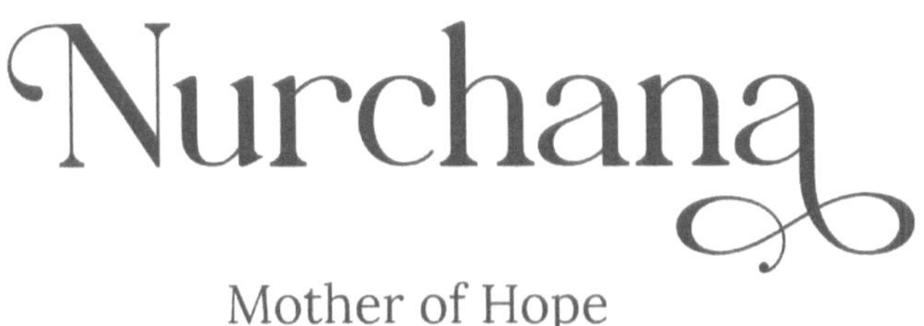

Nurchana

Mother of Hope

DHANANJAY KUMAR

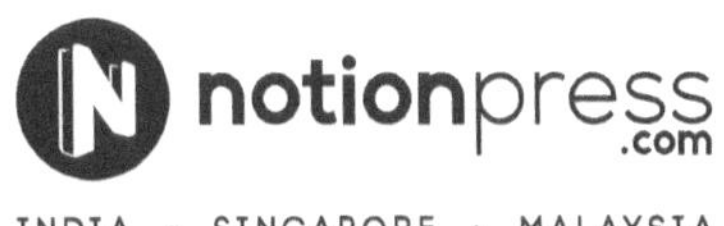

notionpress.com

INDIA • SINGAPORE • MALAYSIA

Copyright © Dhananjay Kumar 2025
All Rights Reserved.

ISBN 979-8-89699-499-2

This book has been published with all efforts taken to make the material error-free after the consent of the author. However, the author and the publisher do not assume and hereby disclaim any liability to any party for any loss, damage, or disruption caused by errors or omissions, whether such errors or omissions result from negligence, accident, or any other cause.

While every effort has been made to avoid any mistake or omission, this publication is being sold on the condition and understanding that neither the author nor the publishers or printers would be liable in any manner to any person by reason of any mistake or omission in this publication or for any action taken or omitted to be taken or advice rendered or accepted on the basis of this work. For any defect in printing or binding the publishers will be liable only to replace the defective copy by another copy of this work then available.

Contents

Contents

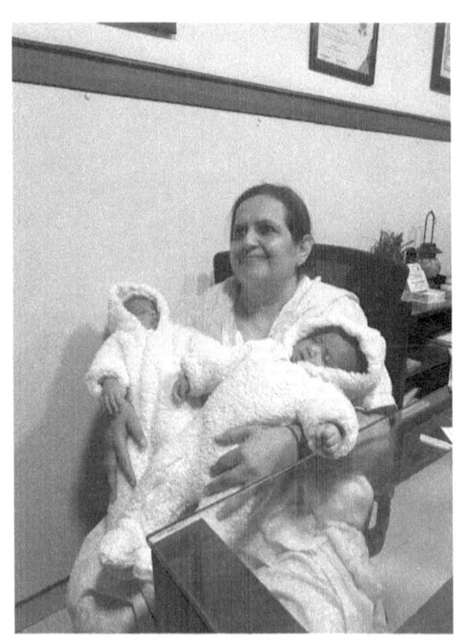

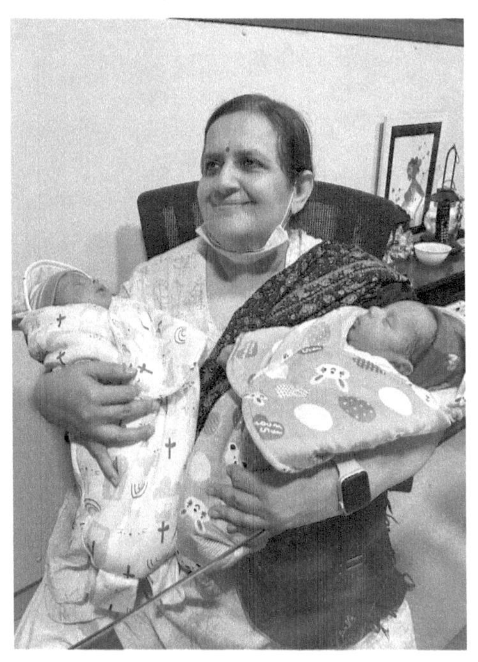

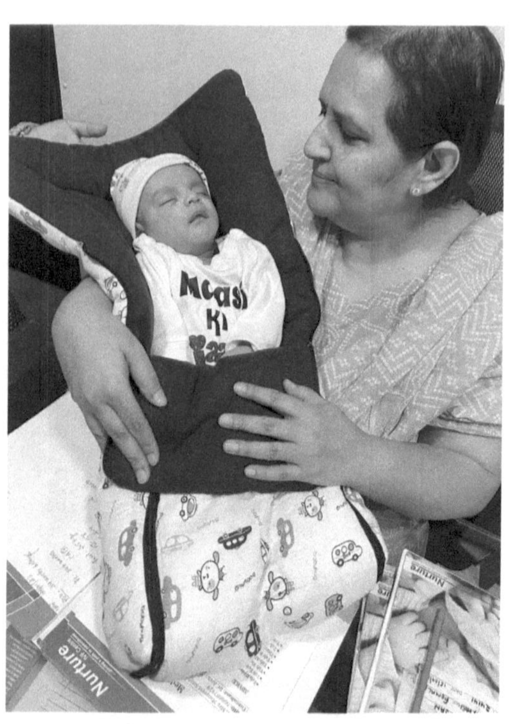

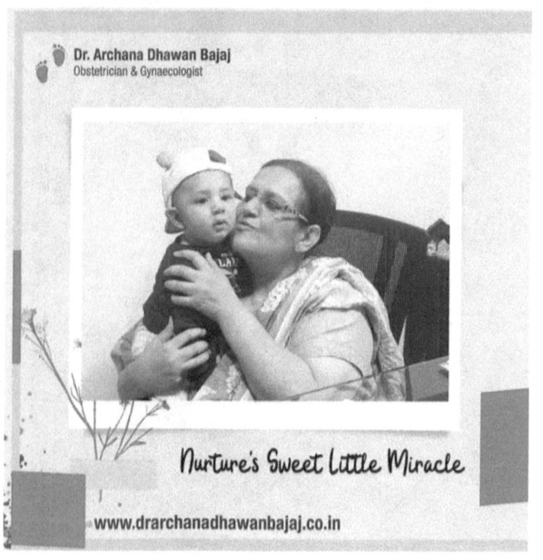
Dr. Archana Dhawan Bajaj
Obstetrician & Gynaecologist
Nurture's Sweet Little Miracle
www.drarchanadhawanbajaj.co.in

Chapter 1

Of Book Born of IVF: A Quest for Excellence

A book is a veritable bundle of pages of joy for a writer and penning it is a veritable labour pain for him. And whenever he runs into writer's block, he experiences a trauma quite akin to that of infertility millions of women under the sun grapple with. A writer can well appreciate the pain of bumps that pop up along process of procreation. The pangs and vicissitudes both experience border on camaraderie.

Nurchana – Mother of Hope is just like my 'take home baby' and brings with it unfathomable happiness that women might feel after having a bundle of joy to fill their desolate houses with squeals. I dedicate this book to hundreds of thousands of childless couples who are toiling day in and day out to take joy to their homes through assisted reproduction technology, IVF (In Vitro Fertilization), a godsend for women who fail to procreate naturally.

The book is a precursor to my forthcoming anthology of best of breed and credible IVF centres under the title 'The Bourn Halls of India', Bourn Hall being the Mecca for assisted fertility centres, the site where 1st test tube baby in the world was born about 46 years ago. The compilation will be part of yet another ambitious project christened 'True Healers', quest for excellences across different specialities. As a health journalist of over two decades in Delhi NCR, most of my times would be consumed by picking holes in healthcare domain to the exclusion of even those centres of excellences that are not only excelling but acquitting themselves honourably and dutifully. But on introspection, I felt there is also a need for affirmative action by way of separating wheat from the chaff and aggregating the best in different specialities so that patients could find genuine healers. This was urgently needed in assisted fertility sphere because there is a clutter of shady facilities dotting every nook and cranny of the country.

While scouting for credible, fecund, genuinely high yielding and go-to assisted fertility centres, I thought to portray one of them as a specimen to my laboured anthology- one that epitomises the gold standard on scale of values. Nurture, IVF centre in Narayana Vihar, which I chanced upon in course of due diligence, merited to be one. This is not at all to suggest that Nurture, with 10,000 and counting IVF babies to its credit so far, is the only exceptionally good IVF centre but only that it is one of the best and genuine centres in the country.

Dr Archana Dhawan Bajaj, presiding over Nurture, made the cut of being a model expert imbibing skills and qualities worth her salt. As a vouched for assisted birthing specialist in India, Dr (Mrs) Bajaj draws bouquets both in home and abroad. On my scale of values, she passed muster and measured up to optimum. Perfection being outcome of a continual process of refinement, especially in medicine, Nurture is well on course striving to ever remain cream of the crop.

Writing a book bordering on hagiography of a private medical facility and its lead doctor is an awkward subject as you face the risk of being branded as writer with benefits. But, with God as witness, I made bold to cross the Rubicon and chose Nurture as my rallying point. I reflected long and hard-days of peeping, watching, eavesdropping, talking - before choosing Nurture as closest to my idea of an ideal assisted birthing facility.

Doctors are always easy meat and liable to be made mincemeat at the drop of a hat, though not completely without reason. Assisted fertility aka IVF, a real deal for multiplying millions of childless couples, is not an exception to it. Of course, lure of lucre has been diagnosed as the dominant motivation in private healthcare sector but there are honest practitioners and conscience keepers in medicine as well and too many at that. They deserve to be given their due.

I carry the conviction that Dr (Mrs) Bajaj exemplifies a very good fertility expert and her 'baby' Nurture is one that optimises towards ideal. This is also my fond hope that this book and my compendium of genuine IVF centres will help childless couples protect themselves from wannabe fertility experts with shady experience. Though it is not easy to sit on judgement, I am not at all conflicted about choosing Dr Archana as my yardstick and epitome.

Besides skills and application of cutting-edge technologies, Nurture fared great on two aspects of overall value system, humanity and ethicality, which in fact became the reason of the centre being chosen by me for the book. These aspects, I think, are critical because unless hope and trust is won in any

IVF facility the chance of taking home baby would diminish greatly because suspicion and stress of a mother to be messes up with skills.

Being blessed with a baby is a matter of intense happiness. A courtyard bereft of chirping of children is a veritable desert of loneliness. As ever widening infertility footprint is taking principle of human procreation in its vice like grip, IVF passes as lighthouse of hope. IVF is priceless- being beyond all manners of mundane prices. Every take home baby is a treasure trove in itself. Measuring an IVF baby by the cost incurred is at best a mean and unkind cut. Joy that emanates after having bundle of joy through IVF is immense and transcends pecuniary consideration.

IVF has come of age and is now well entrenched in the popular imagination of people. Many movies, including box office hits like, Vicky donor and Good News, made around this technology speak a volume about the great purpose it is serving in the society. The population of IVF babies are increasing by the day. As infertility is increasingly widening its net, the success rate is constantly on the increase. Still, this useful process has more often than not been on the receiving end. But shooting the process is not at all desirable. IVF might have degenerated into unconscionable laissez faire in wrong hands and regulation of the sector for sure is called for. Doubtless IVF centres of dubious standard have mushroomed all over the country and unsuspecting childless couples are falling for them and are being duped of their hard-earned money and dreams of bundles of joy.

There are a number of centres of excellence which need to be segregated from the sterile ones.

I hope my anthology 'The Bourn Halls of India' which is in the works, will serve as a ready reckoner of genuine IVF experts for childless couples.

– Dhananjay Kumar

Chapter - 2

Prologue
Diagnosing Genuine Healers Need of the Hour

Medicine is but a sacred calling. There cannot be any 'second opinion' about it but, painfully, it is not so as it is being practised today. The practice is no more as pristine as it was once thought to be. But it does not follow that there is a complete absence of virtue in the domain. There are still a lot of genuine practitioners who are acquitting themselves most honourably. The need of the hour is to insulate them from the slur the profession is generally facing and identify those who have moral worth along with their clinical competence.

It must be acquiesced in a sober fact that healthcare has an underbelly marked by unscrupulous elements and unsuspecting patients are up for grab by them. It is fair to say that the trust deficit between patients and the doctors is at its lowest ebb. Ethicality has taken a back seat and profiteering has muddied the profession once regarded sacrosanct. Nevertheless, thanks to good number of genuine healers, the domain has not turned into an Augean Stable of sort. Therefore, to my mind, painting the entire community of healers in black would be unkindest cut of all. It must be cutting honest practitioners to the quick to see that they are being clubbed with the unconscionable lot.

The book '**Nurchana- Mother of Hope**' by Dhananjay Kumar, a health journalist of over two decades in Delhi NCR, is a beginning in the right direction as it identifies, without mincing words, a healer who largely measures up to his idea of an ideal in medicine. The book is like a whiff of fresh air in the midst of daily dose of stories about sordid side of the vocation. The book is woven around Dr Archana Dhawan Bajaj, an ace IVF and fertility expert and her birthing facility Nurture. I hope one would very much like the sound of Nurchana which is a blend of two solemn words Nurture and Archana. I am cocksure Mr Kumar must have found Dr Archana passing muster both in letter and spirit after due diligence and thorough digging,

By making a name in Health Journalism, Dhananjay, in fact, has done me proud. If I take a word from the theme around which this book has been written, I can well call Dhananjay as my own baby because as Editor in Chief of Nai Dunia in Delhi, I was the one who appointed him as first health editor in India. I am happy to say that Mr Kumar measured up to my expectations from him.

Health writing has long been Dhananjay's province. By embarking on a journey to aggregate true healers across all specialities, he has taken a leap of faith of sorts. It is good that he has decided also to dwell on the bright side of healthcare. I wish in his next book 'Bourn Halls of India' that is already in the pipeline, he will make an exhaustive list of fertility experts who measure up to the benchmark that he has enunciated in this book. As infertility is increasing its footprint in India, true IVF experts are the need of the hour to cater to thousands of childless couples in India despairing for their bundles of joy.

Upward of two decades is a pretty long time for knowing and recognising the milieu one is watching from close quarters. Through these years, Mr Kumar built his reputation as a conscientious health journalist and has emerged as an influencer and key opinion maker in healthcare. He has the advantage of being at a vantage point to rate doctors on scale of values. He has the locus standi to nudge people to his pantheon of true healers. Finding a genuine doctor is really daunting these days as there is a huge trust deficit. In the middle of such scenario, think of a patient who is in complete darkness about whom to go for treatment. Anthology of true healers that Dhananjay has embarked on to write can well do a handholding. Dhananjay by virtue of being health writer for such long time should also be kind of ready reckoner for such patients.

I believe in addition to writing about what ails healthcare, a health journalist's responsibility is also to champion true healers. There is no doubt that ethicality is the mark of a true leader. I do not know much about practice of Dr Archana Dhawan Bajaj but she being in Dhananjay's circle of faith speaks a volume. A journalist's job is not digging up dirt only but also to take affirmative action so that people could choose the right ones. Chosen by Dhananjay as an archetype of a true healer is a huge endorsement for Dr Archana.

If there are women who complain that they have been fleeced of money or duped by false hope selling by wannabe IVF experts, there is a greater number of women too who are eternally indebted to IVF fertility experts for giving them bundles of joy and never tire of showering gratitude and love on them. This book, I think, is more a portrayal of an ideal fertility expert than promoting a particular IVF expert. I would rather readers read this book as benchmarking of a centre of excellence and the specialist presiding over it. I am cocksure Dhananjay must have dug up facts while picking one from among many. It is equally commendable that some centre of excellence should offer itself for scrutiny to a journalist. This much I know, Dhananjay Kumar has so assiduously built and fiercely guarded his reputation and is well in a position to judge a doctor on his scale of values. One fact particularly seems going big in Dr Archana's favour is that she is daughter of an army doctor who forged her in the values he cherished most. Her father was a great healer, the greatest Gynaecologist of his time and a stickler for moral uprightness. As is famously said, an apple does not fall far from the tree; Dr Archana turns a spit image of her illustrious father.

As I hear the PM Modi government has decisively moved to regulate the assisted fertility domain by making an act, it is a right development to clean the practice just as the doctor ordered. The alacrity of PM Modi government to purge the profession that involves millions of women despairing for bundles of joy is highly commendable. This will certainly go a long way in stamping out unscrupulous players from the domain and save unsuspecting couples from being duped.

Padma Shri Alok Mehta

A renowned senior journalist

Chapter 3

The Chosen One: Born to Be

Dr (Mrs) Archana Dhawan Bajaj did not choose her vocation of being a fertility expert of her own. It just happened to her because resolutely and stubbornly brainiac that she is, she was spoilt for choices on her career path and she could have donned an altogether different hat and any she wanted. But after nearly 20 years down the line, she feels it in her bones that she is 'Chosen One' to minister to the needs of thousands of childless couples longing for squeals of bundles of joy in their lonesome homes.

Wishes were indeed horses for Mrs Dhawan on the cusp of choosing her calling and she would ride to at will wherever she set her sights on. She was like 'never underestimate Archana Dhawan in the making'. She had nerve to decide to strive for any goal post you dare to her. Just say to her- this is not for you; she would invariably mutter in her mind- Just you wait! And she would silently be on mission to prove you wrong. In her case, it was like 'she came, she saw, she conquered'. No career seemed out of bound for her, which she amply proved every time she was dared. Her career triumphs were really stuff of a versatile. Sampling her career curve shows how she was stolen for procreation duty from among various competing options quite within her reach.

Dr Archana carries the conviction that she was made for this calling, elected for IVF to nurture motherhood. The smiles on faces of childless couple seem divine to her. As is Dr Archana's wont, she looks every infertility case as a challenge and habitually gives her 100 percent as failure is a word she dreads most, though it cannot be verified whether her intelligence has anything to do with Nurture's high yield of take-home babies- which is over 10,000.

It clearly seems divinity had decided her purpose and passion as assisted fertility expert. The die was cast when Dr Archana was born. In the hindsight, the circumstances of her birth point to the scheme of things she was being fitted into. Scriptures' sacred verse-- Before I formed you in the womb, I chose you: before you came forth from the mother's womb, I consecrated you-- rings quite true in her case. Her birth was eventful and imperceptibly prophetic. As if Maulana Azad Medical College (MAMC) eyed her as its student just as she was born, it happened to be her alma mater in medicine later on and she was delivered by her teacher- to- be. The most prominent Gynaecologist of the time, Dr B G Kotwani, who got her delivered, shaped her formative years in the medical college. Isn't curious coincidence that the hospital where she was born became her medical college and the gynaecologist who delivered her became her guide there?

Reminiscing her medical college days, Dr Archana says, 'It must be written in the stars that I will be a fertility expert. I often felt chosen one for my medical college. I was blessed to have Dr BG Kotwani in my corner as my teacher. Her teaching is an indelible part of my fertility training. I feel privileged to be her student and hold her in highest esteem.'

The vocation of nurturing motherhood is her real calling and seems to have the sanction of divinity. Despite various allurements of other career options, she embraced vocation of bringing joy to women longing for tiny tots. As a fertility expert she feels it was her true north and thanks God for assigning her to it. She discovered her authentic self in this profession. IVF is a combination of her purpose and beliefs. Dr Archana says, 'The smile of couples after having bundle of joy gives me satisfaction to the fullness, I reckon, other calling would not have given me. Then, what could be more satisfying and gratifying than walking the path of my celebrated father under whose wings I learnt to fly and whom I adored for his attributes. I have the force of feeling that I was preordained to engineer joys for lonely homes.' Indeed! Dr Archana is a rare blend of sharp instincts and intelligence.

In fertility domain as well, she showcases the same class- a world class expert of IVF. While nurturing test tube babies she likes the sound of being looked at as mother from all across the globe. She is still the cynosure of the babies she gifted to childless couples coming to Nurture from different countries, especially from Afghanistan. In fact, she turns to be the biggest Delhi exporter of happiness to infertile and childless couples in Afghanistan. As high as 50 couples from Afghanistan, come every month to her clinic Nurture. Dr Archana says, 'working on childless couples from abroad and giving them their gifts for life, I knew motherhood knows no bounds. It is a great feeling that so many children across the world looks at you as mother besides their own. For me nothing is more fulfilling than 'gifting' babies to childless couples who trek all the way from the war-ravaged country to have their bundles of joy.'

As an IVF expert, Dr Archana is perennially in labour pain for couples she treats. Though IVF babies are fertilized on petri dish, she feels as if she bears them all in her own womb because as they mature, she shares the same moments of anguish and hope that their mothers bearing them went through. Dr Archana says, 'It thrills me as my territory of affection and love transcends the artificial borders.'

Though the high numbers take home babies so far is a matter of joy but she undergoes the pangs also of failures as intensely as the real parents. Dr Archana says: "Handing out babies to childless couple is a passion for me. But practising this hope technology has its highs and lows I always happen to alternate between happiness at the success and sadness at the failure. Every failure of the cycle is a personal failure. It is a veritable 'labour pain', so to say." With take home baby success rate reaching 70 percent, a rate only a few IVF centres would match, Dr Archana finds this procedure and the attendant vigil on the maturing baby a very taxing one. Here music comes handy in handling her tense moments. She sings to relax. She is endowed with gift of good voice and learnt singing from a teacher who came to her home to tutor her how to sing.

Dr (Mrs) Bajaj feels particularly subdued by the tenacity of the childless couples to get their bundles of joy. They do not want to leave any 'sperm or ovum' unturned to get the sunshine for their 'empty' homes. The motherly passion is borne out by one of her clients, 33-years-old Mukti, who got blessed with two sons Tejas and Rajas after well over a dozen failed cycles. Think of it: a baby at more than 15 lakh rupees. She is very active on Facebook and flaunts her precious find with gay abandon. On her Facebook she writes— "Dr Bajaj planted seeds of life in me, gifted me two little ones who made my life." Dr Bajaj considers her the greatest trophy of her success in her entire stint of assisted fertility. Dr Bajaj says: "She had 15 failures somewhere else. When she came to me, I tried to convince her that now the only option left was to adopt but she was far from relenting. Two cycles failed in my centre too but as was ordained, she made it in the 18th cycle."

On Mother's Day every year, Dr Bajaj is swamped by letters, SMSs, cards, calls, paintings, flowers, thank you cards bearing touching words like "thanks ma" Some of them call her "*asli* mummy". On the back of her seat in Nurture hangs a very telling painting sent to her from USA by the test tube boy of an NRI doctor. In the painting- There is a baby protruding through the broken corner of the outer covering of an egg. Written overhead is: Thanks Dr Archana Bajaj. She is deluged by grateful missives from far and wide now and then.

Dr Archana sums up saying, 'Regardless of whatever amount of money spent, once a couple gets their bundle of joy, it is always a gift for them. The money spent is nothing compared to the fund of joy they get.' But Dr (Mrs) Bajaj gifts child literally as well. She does it free for some who have no money but only an unfathomable urge for motherhood.

In her practice, Dr Archana comes across many heart warming and touching moments and instances. Recounting them, she reminisces a unique instance- To bring India,

Afghanistan and Pakistan on the same page of love and affection may seem an impossible feat to achieve but Dr Archana has done it with great success. Think of an Afghani lady coming to India to conceive and delivering the baby on Pakistani territory. Is it not a 'love triangle' impossible to think diplomatically? Dr Bajaj delivered this diplomacy on a Petri dish. A young childless Afghani couple; 25-year-old Sufiya with her 35-year-old husband Hamid visited Nurture long ago. Her husband was suffering from zero sperm i.e., Azoospermia. With IVF done at Nurture, Sufia gave birth to a baby boy in Pakistan.

If medicine is as good as a team, she has her IVF facility well nurtured. Dr Archana said, 'It takes a veritable village to craft a baby to be taken home.'

Dr Archana's formative years took smooth with the rough. She says' 'I learnt my life lessons in war like situations. It was as tortuous and uncertain as the attainment of motherhood is. Since her parents were Army doctors and were posted in Jalandhar at the time of her birth, she was taken under the wing of her grandparents who lived in Ludhiana. Her grandfather was an Income Tax officer there. She had her early schooling in Ludhiana. Her grandfather was a huge part of her growing up. On her parents' Allahabad posting, she had the opportunity to study in St Marry School. The fibre of gene she inherited was of top quality. Dr Archana says with elan, 'I belong to an exquisite bloodline and I am proud of my ancestry which was marked by best of values. All of my elders who were in my corner filled me with values that I still hold sacred in my heart. All good values that Nurture stands for ran in my family'

In the gated community of army cantonment, she got steeped in the virtues of Army and was nurtured in values. In crisis time, the head officer will take one for the team. And those virtues became abiding values and got embedded in her mind and never let her go astray.

In Guahati posting, She had the environ of Gated community of Army Cantonment and soaked in the values which define core of Indian Army. Cut off from outside world, winds of communication were slow and tedious. Even connecting to Delhi on phone would take 24 hours. Commanding officer would be looked at as father figure and would earnestly act like one. Dr Archana adds, 'My father was highly respected gynaecologist and well decorated. I can boast my gene was of very good quality. My mother proved a mountain of strength for me and she never let me fall apart in the midst of traumatic events like younger brother suffering from Down syndrome and dying in the prime of his life.'

'My school life was a chequered one. From Ludhiana to Guahati to finally Delhi was a long zigzag entailing twists and turns of disparate terrains. But armed with strict Army upbringing, my mother keeping hawks' eye on me came handy and I could navigate the ups and downs with ease. The quality of upbringing never let me fall apart and despite uneven times, remained in one piece and navigated the domain with ease'

When she came to Delhi, Loretto was her first school where she studied till class 10. It was a school where children of army men and big business men studied. It was a girls' only school and main motto behind sending girls to this school was to make them learn dressing up, etiquettes and impeccable manners, study being secondary. But upbringing kept her on course and always righted her ship. For entrance in Loretto she needed to command Hindi, which she just knew smattering of till then. And lo and behold! just in bare three months in the run up to entrance test, she mastered Hindi. And finally she was a topper in Hindi too. She did it with sheer grit. Again, the usual super Brainiac Archana! Her gifts are without compare among IVF experts. Given the kind of intelligence she showed, it is not hard to imagine she could be top of the crop in any field.

From formative years of schools to carving out career contours, her saga was always picking up the gauntlet and is paved with career conquests. This grain in her made her confront crossroad of her life. She was in an enviable position to decide her career at will. Under her mother's strict upbringing, she earned the tag of an achiever and took her parents and grandparents unawares by her secret goal missions and successes. They just needed to say- not for you baby. 'I will race you' would be retort in her mind. Challenge was an incentive to her and spurred her to act to make it. Or how else one explains she making it to IIT with a very good rank in her first attempt- hole in one indeed! Needless to say, cracking IIT at that time without any coaching was quite something that speaks a volume about her super intelligence. She also aced entrance to DU's St Stephen College, cradle of many a prodigy and big academic guns. It was given that she was tenacious with capital T. In her prime, the time of picking her profession, she had whatever it takes for excellence in any field she might have coveted. She was always driven kind, ahead of the game, never a quitter. Challenge was her steroid. If she decided she could crack any competitive examination and be any somebody- a doctor, an IAS, an engineer and what have you.

There was nothing you could say was not for her. She could have been an engineering genius if she wanted. She was a light under bushel - would not brag, not tell others about her talents and what she was up to till she would pull a rabbit out of the hat- quite something.

Dr (Mrs) Archana says, 'The challenge would invariably fire me up and involuntarily resolve me to respond with vehemence. It was just by a skin of teeth that I became an IVF expert for engineering bundle of joy; I would have been an engineer and might have clawed my way up to the top and would have taken altogether a different path. And, you bet! I would have been an IAS or IPS and whatnots, had I resolved to fulfil the dream of my father about me.' Dr Archana was doubtless a catch the bull by horns type.

In her stint in gated community, there was some Mittal girl whom all girls called Didi. She was role model for them because she had cracked National Talent Search exam. She was Archana's father's favourite. Her father would think Dr Archana did not make the grade for All India Talent Search exam. Though she bonded well with Mittal girl because she was good but the fact that she earned her reputation due to her talent search success cut her to the quick. One day her resolve firmed up. Without announcing it to anyone, she got down to preparing it and to the surprise of all and sundry, made it and got 15th position in the talent search exam.

Dr Archana topping ICSC board and being called by DPS RK Puram, the dream convent school in Delhi for admission finally earned her the tag of achiever. Her grandfather had the opportunity to have tea with DPS principal. Her grandfather was thrilled at this and went to town telling all and sundry how his granddaughter was a prodigy and done him proud. Of course, a guardian sipping tea with DPS principal was a rare treat. DPS was a new phase in her life because it was co-ed school.

Chapter - 4

Learnt from the Best of Class

Dr Archana Dhawan Bajaj is a doyenne in the field of IVF because of the kind of first- rate training she received in course of her quest for excellence in Assisted Reproductive Technology. She did not become the kind of veteran in IVF domain she is today right out of the gate. It was a steep learning curve which lent to her exceptional assisted birthing skills amply corroborated by her high count of take home babies' success rates i.e. a bit shy of 75 percent. She learnt from the best of class. Being abundantly brilliant and sharp, she would get the grip in no time. Her workshops for training happened to be top notch centres of excellences of the world which are talked about with respect even today. She also landed in Sir Ganga Ram Hospital doing DNB there in the company of galaxy of great gynaecologists.

But first thing first- She has a pedigree of obstetrics and gynaecology. Her father Col A K Dhawan himself was highly respected and well decorated gynaecologist of the time from whom she derives her motive to turn her IVF facility Nurture into best of class following the lead of her illustrious late father's dream to establish a birthing centre of the fame of original Bourne Hall in London where first test tube baby in the world was born. Her father has left a kind of legacy as a philanthropist and gynaecologist of first water in Narayana Vihar Dr (Mrs) Bajaj can proudly lean on. She learnt her rope in the veritable company of who's who of assisted birthing.

She picked up the knack of assisted birthing at the feet of some of the best minds of IVF world. In her words, just when she got started she had the good fortune of learning from the 'queens' and all time great fertility doyenne of the time. If she is being able to fill the homes of thousands of childless couples today, there is a sound foundation of training underpinning it. If you take a look at her education graph in chapter named 'The Chosen One', you would know that she is singularly intelligent. In IVF practice, blend of her intelligence and training from best of the minds is leading to her amazing accomplishments in her domain. Her training at the hands of big guns of fertility has made her such a natural in IVF.

Dr (Mrs) Bajaj nostalgically says, 'In Nurture, I am nurturing my Papa's dream. Papa wanted to set up an assisted birthing centre of the grade of original Bourne Hall. Dr Hrishkesh Pai was pioneer in India when Papa was alive and imagining his Indian Bourne Hall. My papa wanted Dr Pai to be CEO of the assisted fertility of his dream.

Queen's Medical Centre of University of Nottingham

This centre in UK was the benchmark of training for assisted fertility. Training here was a must at that time to go to town flaunting one's superiority in assisted birthing. IVF experts use training here as a badge of honor. Dr Archana Dhawan Bajaj did M. Med. Sci in ART of course. But icing on the cake is that Dr (Mrs) Bajaj topped in the course there and the centre referred her to the topmost birthing centre of the time in Jordan for extensive hands on training. The Aman Farah hospital in Jordan received Dr Archana as a royalty because of scintillating performance in Nottingham University.

The M. Med Sci in Assisted Reproductive Technologies at the University of Nottingham was the first and one of the most successful Masters level courses in the UK. It was a famed nursery for embryologists and other professionals in reproductive medicine for UK and many other countries in Europe, Asia, the Middle East and Africa. The Nottingham Masters was a cut above the rest for providing a thorough understanding of the science and core skills needed for assisted conception. It was a huge success and over the years provided much of the senior workforce to the whole world for the reproductive science. Established in 1993, this one year course equipped aspiring scientists and clinicians to enter the growing field of reproductive biology. It equipped graduates with formal theoretical and practical training necessary within this highly specialised discipline. A major feature and strength of the course was that the primary components, in terms of reproductive physiology, research methods, clinical embryology and clinical medicine were all provided by experts who were highly active within their own areas of expertise. Its reputation of being breeding ground of IVF experts can gauged from the fact that when this course was closed, it created a scenario of biggies all over the world crying like babies. Its closure left a real void in assisted fertility domain.

Mecca of assisted fertility in Jordan

Dr Archana Dhawan Bajaj looks at Aman Farah Hospital in Jordan as her Mecca of real training. Its founder Dr Zaid Kilani was the greatest veteran of assisted fertility of the time. Dr (Mrs) Bajaj says, 'Dr Kilani is my role model. Work culture of this hospital and persona of Dr Kilani changed my vision. I learnt dedication and patience needed in IVF from Dr Kilani. He was about 70 year old but I always found him up and doing. Very high volume done in his 7- star hospital there proved a perfect venue for me to sharpen my skills. Dr Kilani was greatly respected all over the fertility domain'.

Farah Woman and Child Hospital is part of Farah Medical Campus specializing in IVF and Genetics, Obstetrics and Gynecology, Fetal Medicine, Neonatal care and Pediatrics. The hospital's legacy includes over 30 years of experience in the field of assisted birthing and is internationally recognized as a centre of excellence for IVF, high risk obstetrics and gynecology. ART unit here is one of the largest worldwide. It serves around 4000 infertile couple a year and is considered to be referral centre for tough cases suffering from repeated IVF failures. The large patient population coupled with excellent success rates led to the ART unit at the Farah hospital to be major attraction for leading infertility centres and pharmaceutical companies worldwide for collaboration in research and development. Dr Archana is truly following in the footsteps of legendary Dr Kilani

In the company of Who's Who in Delhi

Sir Ganga Ram was an iconic birthing centre where all prominent fertility experts and gynaecologists congregated. She did her DNB in Sir Ganga Ram Hospital in 2000. Sir Ganga Ram consisted of a galaxy of gynecologists at that time. The gynecologists there were considered queens of birthing. Dr B G Kotwani, Dr S K Ghai Bhandari (who delivered Congress Leader Rahul Gandhi, his sister Priyanka Gandhi and her two children), Dr Indrani Ganguli, Dr Abha Majumdar (to whom is credited with first IVF baby in North India), Dr Promila Chadda et al. I is a queer coincidence that Dr B G Kotwani, Fellow of Royal College of obstetricians and Gynecologists, FRCOG (London), the most prominent of gynecologist of the time under whom Dr Archana Dhawan Bajaj was born in LNJP also became her teacher in Maulan Medical College and shaped her formative years in the medical College. Again Dr Kotwani was in her corner when she was doing her DNB and had the luck to learn to fly under his wing. Dr Bajaj worked in many high end assisted birthing centers in Delhi and got offers from other centers but soon the dream of her father caught with her and led to establishing her Nurture

Chapter 5

Sanctum Sanctorum of Fertility

Always feeling prayer has become Dr Archana Dhawan Bajaj's second nature through her IVF practice because she makes divinity her witness, every time she enters the sacred chamber to blend sperm and egg on the petri dish and transfer embryo thereafter. Amen is a word sewn intrinsically in her mind. Faith and prayer are abiding elements of her being and are source of her power to calm the storm and the tumult that childless couples harbour in their hearts. This leaning on divinity steadies her own emotional exigencies. Nurture naturally is steeped in sacrament of its presiding deity.

One aspect that clearly emerges is that it is not God versus Medical Science in Nurture, one of the most prolific IVF facilities in India with over 10,000 babies to boast of. Nurture's ecosystem is sublime and confluence of science and spiritualism.

Assisted reproductive science seamlessly blends with spiritualism. As Sanctum Sanctorum is to a priestess, Nurture is to its custodian, leading IVF expert, Dr Archana Dhawan Bajaj. Her first name Archana meaning worship itself sends spiritual vibes and is suggestive of the faith system she is nurtured on. The High Priestess of the assisted birthing technology, Dr (Mrs) Bajaj has religiosity baked into her. It is wisdom from divine that firms up her mental strength. Nurture derives its sanctity from Dr (Mrs) Bajaj's unshakeable faith in divine scheme of things. It is a happy coincidence that the name of the place Narayana Vihar where Nurture stands in its glory and grandeur echoes divinity.

Religiosity is intrinsic to Dr Bajaj's being. It is befitting for the vocation because many Studies too have found that spiritualism is an enabling element in IVF journey. Spiritualism has been bequeathed to Dr (Mrs) Bajaj by her parents as she being named as Archana amply shows. True to her name, she follows the dictum- Work is Worship. This self-effacing has rid her of ego that might have crept into her being due to her flawless fertility wisdom. IVF for her is vocation, not profession. Submission to God has been disciplining factor in her journey as IVF expert. The impressive figure of birth of over 10,000 IVF babies might have gone into head of any IVF expert but Dr (Mrs) Bajaj is quite untouched by hubris of any kind. This is the natural corollary of her faith in the almighty.

Despite high end training and remarkable IVF success, Dr (Mrs) Bajaj's humility transcends her sterling skills. Steeped in religiosity, she is far from God complex and attributes birth of every IVF baby in Nurture to God, the ultimate procreator above. She says 'I remember God every time eggs and sperms are blended on Petri Dish.' For her, every attempt at IVF is a leap of faith and Divinity helms the birth of every baby, regardless of the process that happens. Birth of a baby is a miracle of God, no matter how that happens. Petri Dish for

Dr (Mrs) Bajaj is like bowl of worship. Mrs Bajaj looks at her profession of procreation as spiritual testament.

Dr Archana Dhawan Bajaj views IVF as godsend and feels she is doing Almighty's work and is his assistant in procreation. To her, performing a job or task that is intended to help others or advance a cause is God's work. We are all committed to doing His work by reaching out to those who need help giving birth to children. IVF technology is in essence a way to help childless couples, the cost is nothing compared to gift of joy that emanates from birth of a baby through IVF. She strongly believes infertility is not at all a curse but it is a goal set by God for some couples and medical science. Some get bundles of joy as a natural gift from God and some have to earn it- with patience and perseverance coupled with assisted birthing techniques.

Dr Archana says she often witnesses Mother of God moments through her vocation as unbelievable and unexpected dots her IVF journey. She feels divinity helps her whenever she finds herself at her wit's end. She assigns utmost success of Nurture, to power presiding universe. She feels her faith in divinity is her sheet anchor and helped her many a time on the rough road of assisted fertility practice. For her, a woman's face lit by bundle of joy in her lap is a vision of God. Children are His legacy. God has always blessed procreation. Faith and religion are intrinsic to Dr Mrs Bajaj's thought processes.

Many studies have found these aspects of spirituality plays a positive role in the outcome of IVF process. They help both fertility doctors and childless couples seeking babies. Those studies have found significant increase in fertilization, high quality embryo and pregnancy rate among couples steeped in religiosity. Couples who included the infertility diagnosis and treatment in their prayers showed an increased pregnancy rate. The high-quality embryos rate was increased among patients who believed that their faith contributed to their decision to undergo infertility treatment. Belief in treatment success positively influenced the embryo quality. The findings in many studies suggest that spirituality plays a role in fine-tuning an infertile patient psychologically.

Mrs Bajaj holds the view that IVF to be effective involves a holistic care which constitutes not only the psychological, social and cultural but religious and spiritual needs as well. Positive religious and spiritual beliefs help childless couples to cope with crisis, and to find meaning and hope in their IVF journey.

Dr Archana Dhawan Bajaj deeply believes IVF babies are God's bonanza showered on humanity. God uses IVF experts to accomplish his purpose. For her IVF is a journey paved in prayer. According to her all children are from God. IVF babies are knit together by the grace of God. Every child is a gift from God regardless of whether he sends it naturally or is conceived medically through IVF and other fertility treatments. Her deep spiritual being knows only God brings humans into being. The union of egg and sperm is an event under benign eyes of Divinity, IVF experts are merely means to that end. In her heart of hearts, she thanks God for every take home baby.

Various studies have concluded devout mothers to be have fewer symptoms of depression and anxiety and have better ability to cope with stress. However, negative religious beliefs namely thinking infertility could be the god's wrath has been found to be linked with harmful outcomes, including higher rates of depression. Dr (Mrs) Bajaj disabuses couples of such negative beliefs and creates a buffer against such negative thoughts. She says negative beliefs such as infertility being God's punishment makes journey of motherhood through assisted birthing tough. Seeing God as punitive is not helpful. According to Dr Bajaj childless couples having loving and kind perception of God are better equipped for IVF journey.

Dr (Mrs) Bajaj makes religion as enabling, not an inhibiting element in IVF odyssey. She feels many a time some paranormal power guides her in IVF. She also thinks her late father is lighting her path from above and she acts accordingly. This link steadies her boat whenever it is rocked by sudden daunting events. Her instincts are laser sharp due to religiosity of her thoughts.

Various studies have concluded prayers helped women get pregnant, naturally or through assisted processes. Research at Columbia University and Cha Hospital of Korea claimed that women undergoing in vitro fertilization had higher rates of pregnancy when groups of strangers anonymously prayed for them. In fact, both self-prayer and the direct support of a religious community have been shown to improve outcomes. Researchers opine that religious factor influence mental and physical health by altering brain function, shifting hormone levels and boosting the immune system.

Researchers were amazed to find that women who were prayed for ended up with a significantly higher pregnancy rate than those who were not prayed for. They claim to have found about 50 percent got pregnant in the prayer group and about 26 percent in the non-prayer group, the study appears in the Journal of Reproductive Medicine. Lead author initially hesitated in publishing their findings, since the results seemed so unlikely. Yet the findings were so statistically overwhelming, the research team decided to share them. Researchers took up the study out of curiosity, and because it had not been done before. And lo and behold, what they found was from out of the world.

Chapter 6

Inseminating Hope

Hope is the only bee that makes honey without flowers

In Nurture, hope is born the day an infertile couple enters its precincts. Hope is a sine qua non for IVF to reach its fruition. Dr Archana Dhawan Bajaj, a name to reckon with in assisted fertility domain, turns a kindred spirit to all childless couples, sheet anchor for floundering emotions of every one of them, striking instant bond. Here Hope is the primal insemination that paves the way for happy denouement of taking home joy.

As success rate is constantly going north and the process is being continually refined and perfected, hope has got a long rope in Nurture. There is hope in the air here and infertile couples do not lose it early.

Though success rate of IVF in Nurture has reached well over 70 percent and has the distinction of being cradle to over 10 thousand bundles of joy, each IVF cycle is a cliff hanger. And clinging to hope is a must for crossing infertility cliff. The womb that reels under suspicion and fear of failure is not fit to hold the delicate sprout transferred there from Petri dish. The first step in the process of In Vitro Fertilization (IVF) is to lift the spirit of motherhood seeking women who might be in the depth of despair. Dr (Mrs) Bajaj and her equally motivated team embody qualities which instil hope and faith, the twin angels which chaperone an infertile woman to motherhood.

Nurture is not a factory; it is a feeling and health workers here are not assembly line workers- at every step childless couples find an affable someone to greet and hold hand. It is a coherent whole steeped in same spirit of empathy. Dr (Mrs) Bajaj has constituted her team in her own image- genial, kind and sincere. She says, 'I have tried my best to create an intimate, holistic kind of experience in Nurture. The ecosystem in an assisted fertility centre is very crucial and must be put together keeping in mind the sensitiveness involved in IVF. Sweet reasonableness is called for to infuse in them a sense of belonging. Overall environment should feel like an oasis in the parched land of infertility'

Navigating cross currents of unhinging emotions with equanimity is Dr Bajaj's strong suit. Over time, she has learnt to transcend her own turmoil while dealing with gut wrenching travails of infertile women. Her job is cut out for her whom she renders with calmness of mind. At first encounter, initiating a conversation with infertile woman is the critical part. The initial impression on infertile couples in an IVF facility is the most important juncture for the quality of IVF journey till end. There is a need first to rid them of accumulated anguish. The seeds of hope have to be sown at the first meeting. Dr (Mrs) Bajaj with her sweet gaze and soft voice clinches triumph over them. She efficiently tackles sob stories and pathos of the moment. She prepares couples to endure the turmoil in their hearts. Dr Archana has heart of gold and she tries her best to feed heart and soul of infertile couples.

In the midst of chaotic emotional ebb and flow, Dr Archana Dhawan Bajaj has an uncanny knack of pacing herself. She faces daily dose of tough moments but undaunted, she maintains her composure and keeps Budhha laughing ever and never lets negative thoughts give a sinking feeling. With her serene look and smiling mien, she survives the giant waves of emotions. Her bedside manners are of highest quality which keeps up the motivation intact. Dr Archana empathises with motherhood seekers as a fellow traveller. Sometimes she finds herself caught up in the moment but fleetingly, she pulls herself together. Dr Archana has a flair for touching the positive chord of childless women.

Dr (Mrs) Bajaj, whose middle name is optimism, is well versed in sowing hope which is the lifeblood for IVF to be successful. She says, 'keeping hope afloat through the process is of course an enabling state of mind but equally important is to know how to manage hope by inculcating positive attitudes towards reality. Unqualified hoping up, where odds are heavily stacked against the prospect of motherhood, is not my way.'

Sample feelings of Delhi's 36 year old Pallavi (name changed), an infertile woman who has come to Nurture after three failed cycles elsewhere. All her efforts and spend of hard-earned money was a bust. She perhaps fell for some dubious fertility centre. Waiting for her turn in Nurture, she says- 'I looked at infertility as bane of my existence. Pursuing pregnancy has left me a fertility junkie and has consumed my conjugal life. We felt like stuck on fertility treadmill. My marriage is a wreck. But many tears later, hope is alive again thanks to Nurture. Unlike earlier fertility centre where I met with a disappointment, Nurture presents a different positive ambience that has raised hopes in me.

Pallavi says further- 'Dr (Mrs) Archana has assumed the role of my kindred spirit. I soon felt the resonance between us. She around makes me feel calmer. I experience instant sense of relief as I cannot help feeling I have found another soul who knows and understands me. She has brought me in touch with certain wisdom. Her ways of looking at things have done me a world of good. She is my cheer leader by helping me continue pursuing my passions and life purpose. I felt we know each other well the moment we met or soon after. I have the feeling of 'I know you' whenever I see her. She has proved a wonderful support system in my life. I feel I can count on her. Dr Archana first told me not to kick myself up for infertility. She impressed upon me that infertility is not anger of God thrust upon me and restored my faith. She has tremendous power of persuasion. I am hopeful of taking a baby from here, maybe I get twin. I am hopeful my 'archana' will be answered in Nurture? The gentle gaze of Dr Bajaj has enlivened my fading hope' Pallavi's tired look glistens while saying all this.

Disabusing infertile women of despair is an art which Dr (Mrs) Bajaj has mastered over time. Her essential goodness of being coupled with this art morphs into a soothing effect.

With strides in advancement in IVF technology, in large number of cases it is peaches and cream these days but real tough is to deal with women who come after failed cycles elsewhere. Dr Bajaj delves right into their eyes to quieten their frayed emotions. To them Dr Bajaj becomes a friend that makes them smile. Dr Archana has the art of going into the soul of woman and embalming the tormented heart. She has such a way with putting thoughts that calms the mind of child seekers instantly. Her soft voice has a unique tranquil ring to it. She builds infertile women up with kindness and sympathetic ear. Words clothed in softness are her devices to calm the mind. She tries to heal the broken hearted and bandage their wound first. Her stirring persuasion sends roots to parched land the childless couple feel like. Some of them are in depths of despair. First thing needed is to soar hope.

Dr (Mrs) Bajaj says, 'I would acquiesce in a sober fact that it is a daunting task and takes us long to disabuse them of their despair. It is the first crucial step. We meet different levels of despair.'

Dr (Mrs) Bajaj constantly alternates between triumph and failure. One can imagine how tough it might be for her to cope with continuous onslaught of diverse emotions. It is a continuous saga of highs and lows for high priestess of procreation. She subsumes in her frail frame all the anguish and trauma of struggle that journey of pregnant mother entails. She is, so to say, in an eternity of labour pain- all rolled into one. For her, Nurture is ride of her life. She is forever on roller coaster trip. She wears the cross for them and endures heart wrenching stories of women craving for motherhood.

She is expected to smile even when she is incapable of smiling. Dr Archana is emotionally invested in every womb and feels her own labour pain. She fiercely guards the sprout in every pregnant womb as if it is her own. But hold on, when it comes to compliance to instructions and regimen regarding IVF process, she is a hard task master and does not hesitate giving them dressing down either.

Dr (Mrs) Bajaj says, 'Ache of being infertile is past all bearing. Labour pain may be excruciating but not being able to bear this pain is far more agonising. They pine for 'pleasurable' labour pain. In such agonised state of mind, hope is a cushion they need most. It is a must for unmitigated success of IVF. Hope improves the odds of fertilization in IVF and vice versa. Sweet nectar will come only if hope is alive. Stress and hopelessness may become the undoing of urge and efforts to get bundle of joy.'

'I witness them from close quarter and cannot remain untouched by the ebb and flow. At every failure, the couple feel as if a giant wave crushed over them. They are swamped by sadness but the real tough is to act strong. The pain of hearing bad news is overwhelming. When infertile women know about the failure of cycle, they feel their knees to buckle, crumpled in a heap of despair. I keep seeing many a face crumbling and trembling after hearing the news of failed cycle. It is at this juncture a fertility expert has the toughest task to sustain the hope. Sometimes, I am caught up in the moment but have to recover for the sake of them. Being carried away with their agonies is a luxury fertility expert can ill afford. The challenge is to keep that pain of failure from crushing them. Bottling up feelings can make things harder. Every day I have to face infertile women down in mouth - unhappy and dejected- in low spirit and my job is to provide them with 'pick-me-up' hope.

Dr Bajaj adds, 'IVF is an emotional and often protracted journey. It is a physical process; they have to undergo a lot of hormones racing through their bodies. It is the emotional ups and downs that are hard. IVF is where hope and fear maintain eternal strife and fleeting joy inspire lasting doubt and we question most what we most desire. The difficulty of IVF is the hope and the shattered hope, the dream that it might happen this time and it does not happen. It is of course a struggle but worth the salt. IVF is a testament to undying hope in the face of heart break after heart break.'

Hope is very important but managing hope is equally important. It is a major challenge during infertility treatment. Some patients work very hard to remain positive and nurture hope, while there are others who are always on nerves triggered by negativity. People in both groups attain healthy pregnancies. And, unfortunately, there are members in both groups who meet repeated disappointments. Managing hope is even more challenging when it comes to looking beyond a specific cycle and the question of when enough is enough. During infertility treatments, there are people who remain hopeful when odds are against them and others who lose hope when test results and medication responses seem promising. But hope is always a desirable element in IVF.

Dr Archana says, 'Enkindling hope is alright but a genuine IVF expert should never lose sight of realism and never stoop to hoping up in cases where prospect is very bleak. To give false hope is plain cruel. I try my best to reconcile optimism and realism. I state frankly the prognosis where there is need to. A balance between optimism and realism is a must.

Summing up, IVF is quintessentially a hope technology and has aptly been named so. The quest of fertility can be emotionally strenuous and demanding. One study concludes that women with infertility felt just as anxious and depressed as women with cancer, hypertension or other co morbidities. Men undergo less emotional upheavals than women do. But given many treatment options for infertility today, even in case of a difficult fertility diagnosis, hope has a chance. Only that infertile couples need to persevere and keep up patience. IVF experts opine that there are many assisted reproductive technology (ART) options for couples who have trouble getting pregnant naturally.

In a credible fertility facility, during IVF process, there is a whole team of physicians, psychologists, embryologists, nurses, and other health professionals who are dedicated to helping the couples have a baby. It is important to manage emotions in a healthy way during infertility treatment. For many infertile women, expressing their anxieties to their partner, family, or friends can help. Couples may also benefit by joining a local infertility support group or seek counselling during treatment. Though the process can be hard to maintain healthy habits when stressed, exercising regularly can be a significant stress buster. Hope should sustain till exhaust of all options available. IVF can be used in conjunction with other ART techniques. Success rates are constantly on the increase. It is all the reason that couples should not lose hope early.

IVF can be an extremely effective way for infertile couples to get pregnant. As doctors continue to refine and perfect IVF techniques, hope has a long lease now. Couples should talk to their doctor about their best treatment options for infertility. But the choice of a credible fertility centre is a must to give hope a chance.

Chapter 7

Nurturing Moral Excellence

As is very rightly said apples do not fall far from the tree, Dr Archana Dhawan Bajaj is natural in morality as she has inherited her molecules of virtues from her father who was epitome of all good values in personal and professional lives. Taking a leaf out of lexicon of fertility, it can well be said Nurture is a surrogate pregnant with good values that Dr (Mrs) Bajaj's father cherished in his life and vocation.

The moral question is not skin deep but intrinsic to Dr Archana's being. Her father Col AK Dhawan being in Indian Army- highly respected and well decorated- Dr (Mrs) Bajaj's core is soaked in the values that permeate and nurture the grand birthing facility. Her probity as a fertility (IVF) expert is deeply rooted in her upbringing. Any deviance from ethical practices is a contraindication in Nurture and malpractice is off limits. The trust and the feeling of being safe within precinct of Nurture is what make it one of its kind.

Dr (Mrs.) Bajaj got her moral fabric woven from values that constitute the ecosystem of Indian army. Those are abiding values in Nurture as a center of excellence of IVF. The values that are baked into someone's being in formative years endure throughout one's life and that is the case with Dr (Mrs) Bajaj who is a stickler for ethics in Nurture. Her moral compass has the indelible imprint of values of her father in particular and that of army in general. Her father being a renowned gynecologist in the army, he had envisioned a fertility center. Nurture being a tribute to his vision, it embodies all principles that he cherished. The moral excellence of Nurture is written in stone and bears signature of Dr Archana Bajaj's hero, her father. In fact, the lineage that she is part of is in single file so far as moral values are concerned. Dr Archana's mother is a spit image of her father and feels pride in the fact that her daughter is walking in the footsteps of her late husband.

Vindicating the saying 'like father like daughter', she is trying utmost to fill in her illustrious father's shoes in terms of probity which keeps her from worldly wise environment wherein ethics are taking back seats. When her father, a profoundly decent man, died there was an unprecedented groundswell of people to give him a grand and epic send off. It was a genuine testimony to generosity of his spirit. Police had to be called in to stem the tide of people milling for his farewell. As if it was not enough to prove his philanthropy and kind heartedness, patients would later on turn up to pay the fees they owed to him. He endeared all people in the locality. For him patients came first, fees later- no matter if someone did not have money to pay. The people in the locality still fondly remember his generosity as a doctor and a man. He even went out of his way to help poor and hapless patients. The stories of his generosity abound in the area. But God called him home very early at the age of bare 42 leaving his extended family of blood and bond inconsolable for a long time to come. His untimely departure for heavenly abode was a great loss to those patients who had no one to turn to.

In the midst of unconscionable laissez faire rampant all around, virtues are becoming scarce commodity in every department of life and to shun lure of lucre is not easy in today's world. But those for whom virtues are a legacy, they are still holding the ground. Dr (Mrs) Bajaj is one such torchbearer of her parental values and takes them straight to her calling. Nurture's moral excellence is transmitted from her great parental legacy. Dr (Mrs) Bajaj is never in a moral quandary and invariably goes for what is right and conscientious. The conscience that she has inherited always guides her to right direction. It is not merely following rules set by the powers that be; the pledge is more than that. Dr Archana is implementing her father's ideals through Nurture. Dr Archana sees Nurture as memorial to her father's value system. The value system that has nurtured Dr Archana Dhawan Bajaj is her supreme inheritance from her late father. Her father's magnanimity, integrity, purity of purpose, commitment to the cause is all stuff she has derived her value system from. Her father's moral code is hers. Her father was a man of great conviction. Protecting something that her father held sacred is her holy grail.

Dr Archana says, 'I feel my father is a guiding spirit over Nurture and have felt many a time, that he is literally guiding me in IVF cases. My instincts are sharp. I find myself awake at the dead of night and feel to intervene in a pregnant woman in a certain way and to my great surprise it turns out that it was perfectly right thing to do. I feel some spirit is moving me for sure.' Trust is when you feel safe with someone. The same spirit keeps Nurture moving.

Dr Archana says, 'I embraced many lessons from Army life. The biggest was lesson of cohesion. This was the time of upbringing when I had vision of virtues of army life. How you live for community? – I learnt from the gated community of Army Cantonment. Outstanding Army culture shaped my way of life. My father was assigned the management of Army mess as Secretary which speaks a volume about my father's integrity and honesty. Getting this post in army is quite something. Under his vigil, no one ever dared to mess with its book.'

Rounding off, Dr Archana says with a tone of finality, 'wherever papa was in the military service or in private practice, he commanded enormous respect due to his purity of purpose and large heartedness. I consider it a great inheritance and will give the world to perpetuate it. Paltry money that comes through immoral means is garbage for me I will not touch it even with a barge pole.' It is this inheritance that gives her unwavering voice in favor of strict regulation to stem unethical practices in IVF domain.

Dr Archana has always been on the front as befits an offspring of military man of honor to demand banishment of unethical practices from assisted fertility. She is champion of globally accepted ethical practices in all manners of fertility treatment. Whenever question of ethical practices arose, Dr Archana spoke her mind without mincing words and never held brief for crass commercialization shunning ethics. On ethical front, Dr Archana is perfect 10. When issue of IVF being done on old couple aged over 70 came up and became a cause celebre, Dr Archana was upfront in criticizing this. She had said, 'I strongly recommend that the ART should not be made available to women below the age of 18 and above the age of 45. IVF at advanced ages come with risks of pregnancy loss, fetal anomalies, stillbirth, and obstetric complications. It is also associated with medical co-morbidities in mother like hypertension, diabetes and heart problems. It poses risks to both mother and child.'

Birthing is a divine and sacrosanct process where a life takes shape. IVF technique is a god send for infertile couples and is increasingly becoming indispensable as infertility widens its footprint. Over 42 years after this hope technique came into being in the middle of controversy, about 10 million IVF babies are dotting the world today. Over 5 lakh mothers take home baby every year. The expert of this birthing technique dons the role of God, the creator of everything under the sun. The IVF expert and facility is expected to look at it as pious process and deliver service as God would do. But sadly enough, the scenario is not above board. Many facilities make this process only means of profiteering. Unethical practices take many a form and the unsuspecting couples fall easy prey to their shenanigans.

Claims of Success rate are largely phony and a large number of couples fall for inflated success rate. Though with advancement, success rate has reached 70 percent but is not evenly applicable on age groups. This is a mark selected birthing facilities have attained. The success rate in birthing couples in their twenties is way different from that of couples in their forties. But while flaunting success rate, many facilities blur this distinction. The difference between conception rate and take-home baby rate must be factored in while determining the success rate. Conception rate is not success rate per se. Conception rate refers to the number of cases where the couple successfully conceives through this assisted process. However, not all of these conceptions result in live births. Conception rate flaunted as success rate create a false hope of higher chance of having a baby and becomes means of duping infertile couples.

Claiming erroneous high success rate to scout for new patients is the number one rampant unethical practice here. Exchanging samples of sperms, eggs, embryos to pull off high success rate, wrongly advising IVF even if it is not indicated just to extract more money, using, even selling embryos or sperms without permission, maintaining no documentation, et al- the list is long. Talk of regulating the assisted birthing practices is often heard but unconscionable practices are on with impunity. Due to such black sheep in the domain, going through IVF turns frustrating, futile and exorbitant for a large number of hapless childless couples. Many of them who even after years of getting pumped with hormones and getting their hard-earned money going up in smoke end up without having the bundles of joy. Such shady IVF facilities are good only on their websites and social media feed. They use manipulated data to attract desperate couples. Those IVF facilities who shun such practices and have genuinely achieved high success rate want this Augean stable cleaned forthwith because they feel their reputation too suffer from collateral damage.

As infertility increasingly escalates, IVF promises to be a light house for childless couples. The global IVF market is pegged at upward of $15 billion. The consistent advancements in the techniques might make it a preferred mode of birthing in the future. As IVF becomes norm rather than exception, there is urgent need for transparency and sound regulation to save this hope technology from ignominy that unethical practices might inflict on it. IVF facility like Nurture serves as standard bearer.

Chapter 8
Thousands Awards & Counting

If awards and honours are counted in terms of mundane trophies, medals, orders, decorations, recitations, plaque, belt, badge, cups et al, even hundreds might sound a hyperbole but if one marks the words spoken by ace cricketer Virendra Sehwag about Dr (Mrs) Archana on the occasion of one such big time honour bestowed on her in London, they are really in thousands and counting.

Virender Sehwag wrote on twitter- 'Congratulations to Dr Archana Dhawan Bajaj for being an inspirational leader. These awards are just a small recognition for her exemplary services.' Coming as it does from an iconic cricketer like him; it really goes for six for Dr (Mrs) Bajaj. Mr Sehwag is spot on as Dr Bajaj is a true and credible IVF expert and a genuine achiever will feel the same way. As IVF is more a vocation for her than profession despite extensive training and acquiring special skills, Dr Archana's greatest award and trophy is a baby that she hands to a childless couple to make a happy home.

Though Dr Archana Dhawan Bajaj has bagged many classy awards and honours and is reckoned as big-league achiever in her vocation, the awards that really thrill her and make her feel special lie elsewhere numbering thousands- over 10 thousand to be precise- which is the number of take-home babies that her birthing centre can boast of. The day her IVF procedure reach fruition, it is her occasion of being awarded. She feels swamped by honours every day of the year as Nurture's babies all over the world consistently adore her.

For ace IVF and fertility expert Dr Archana Dhawan Bajaj, the greatest trophies are those test tube babies her world class advanced Fertility centre Nurture has so far produced. They are many scattered in different parts of the world, giving her the tag of Mother Unlimited.

It is not to say that the formal awards that are given to her are of no value. Some of them make authentic statements on the calibre of the recipients. Dr Archana Dhawan Bajaj has the distinction of getting many high-end awards and she respects them all and feels privileged to have them.

One such award that Dr (Mrs) Bajaj is recipient of is Global Asian of The Year Award in Singapore. It is undoubtedly a huge one and big time, counted among very prestigious one. It underlines an accomplishment of a great value. Dr Bajaj, the benign baby and mommy maker, was bestowed the Global Asian of The Year Award 2016 on January 24, 2017 in Singapore. Mrs Bajaj was among the Asia's 70 brands and leaders to get one of the most prestigious global awards given every year by highbrow magazine Asia one.

All the recipients of Global Asian of The Year Awards were short listed on the basis of extensive public survey and points given by jury. Some of the notables who got this award with her were Kamini Rao of Milan IVF centre, Dilip Surana, CEO of Microlab, Dr Minnie Bodhanwala and Vikram Nayar, Singaporean parliamentarian of Indian Origin.

Dr Bajaj says, 'It pleased me to get this award with veritable Who's Who from diverse fields but my moment of utmost fulfilment comes every time I hand out a baby to a childless couples. For every one of them, I invest my passion for giving joys to them.

Dr (Mrs) Bajaj loves the filial feeling of global motherhood. Childless couples coming from countries UK, Australia, Iran, Iraq, Dubai, Nigeria, Afghanistan, Pakistan, Nepal and Bangladesh et al got their bundles of joy in Nurture under her motherly care. Dr Bajaj is still avidly remembered by those test tube babies as mom. Though surrogacy has been almost banned in India Dr Archana Dhawan Bajaj is credited with birth of many bundles of joy through surrogacy too but icing on the cake is that, even in the midst of raging talk of exploitation of surrogate mothers, she is still adored by women who rented their wombs to childless couples via her centre. Those surrogates still feel indebted to Dr Bajaj because surrogacy and money that come with it had transformed their lives. She ensured that they are given their due and much more. For Dr Archana, it should be a lifelong relationship of indebtedness of childless couples to women renting their wombs for the birth of their bundles of joys.

Dr Archana says, 'love and respect keep streaming in to me all year round from them from all over the world through letters, SMSs, calls, paintings, flowers, cakes, thank you cards bearing heart-warming words.' Dr Archana Dhawan Bajaj has emerged as the biggest exporter of joy to infertile couples of over 15 countries.

The tiara conferred on her in London, the mecca of assisted birthing, after Singapore is another one that makes her a cut above the rest. These constitute the awesome twosome for ace IVF prima donna Dr (Mrs) Bajaj.

The one in London makes it a glory on a trot. Measuring up to this, thanks to her impeccable assisted birthing credentials, was a kind of leap of faith for her. In the star studded 'The Oval', Dr. Bajaj was conferred the coveted title of 'Inspirational Leader of New India' on May 12. The 'Grande Dame' of IVF got the tag in the presence of international luminaries from across the globe. The praise of Dr (Mrs) Bajaj by world class cricketer Virendra Sehwag for this award packed a punch in the value of the award for her. Virendra Sehwag, congratulating her on this award, said- these awards are just a small recognition for her exemplary services.

Dr. Bajaj's assisted birthing and IVF centre, 'Nurture' in Delhi (Narayana), widely appreciated for ethical surrogacy, has earned the tag of being a veritable 'Bourn Hall' of India. The ice on the cake is that she got this award in the vicinity of legendary and original IVF centre Bourn Hall in London where first test tube baby of the world had seen the light of the day in the hoary past.

As always, humility took the better of Dr. (Mrs) Bajaj on the ecstatic occasion. Just after receiving the coveted honour, she was a picture of modesty as always. Dr. Bajaj said, 'I am not sure how deservedly the feather rests on my cap. For me in fact, no award is as valuable as when I hand over a baby to a childless couple. That in fact is the greatest trophy for me and I have gotten it many a time in my test tube baby birthing career so far. Yes, I find this award in London a little flattering because getting it in neighbourhood of fabled Bourn Hall' is whale of an honour.'

Center for International Competitiveness and Research launched the glittering annual *Global Power Brands* compendium along with the mega listing of the *World's Most Recognizable Brands*. The launch was presided over by legendary cricketers Alec Stewart (former captain of the English cricket team) and Kumar Sangakara (one of the greatest Sri Lankan ODI players). The awardees included doyens of diverse field including professors from Oxford. In medicine, Dr Bajaj turned out to be single in the Oval Hall of fame.

Arindam Chaudhuri, the founder of Power Brands, gave the inaugural speech outlining the need for global humanism through a more equal world. The inductees into the *Power Brands Hall of Fame* also included Nobel Laureate Leymah Roberta Gbowee, Member of Parliament Mark Durkan, iconic Sri Lankan cricketer Kumar Sangakkara and leading Indian tycoon Pankaj Munjal. The annual international brands' research is undertaken on tens of thousands of brands from multiple industry segments across the globe.

Being chosen for World Women Leadership Congress Award too speaks a volume about her standing among IVF specialists. But she is far from resting on her laurels. She is seamlessly nurturing her passion for giving happiness to childless parents by handing them bundles of joy.

What Asia One, the prestigious magazine, bestowing award on her, wrote on Dr Archana Dhawan Bajaj also constitutes a veritable award. It has not rained but poured praise on her. The magazine has called Dr Archana and rightly so – The Messiah with A Mission. The article is being reproduced here as it is

The Messiah With A Mission

Spreading smiles and bringing joys to the despair-clad families of childless couples, Dr Archana Dhawan Bajaj, a renowned IVF Expert, is consistently turning the dreams of umpteen aspiring parents of getting their bundles of joys to reality, through her clinic 'The Nurture IVF' **BY RICHA SANG**

Armed with qualifications such as an MBBS, DNB, MNAMS and M. Med Science in Assisted Reproductive Technology from the University of Nottingham, UK, Dr Archana Dhawan Bajaj has dedicated her life towards serving the humanity with her hard work and possesses a never ending determination to bring a positive change in the lives of her patients both in India and Abroad. Offering smiles to hundreds of couples the world over, aspiring to pave their path to parenthood, Dr Bajaj has received training from renowned centres like Nurture IVF centre (Nottingham, UK) and Farah IVF specialist centre and Hospital (Jordan). Through her unceasing ambition to excel, she has gained expertise in reproductive endocrinology, Infertility, Assisted Reproductive Technology (ART), High Risk Pregnancy Management, Laparoscopic Surgeries and Hysteroscopic Surgeries (Minimal Invasive Surgeries).

Specialized To Succeed

Gaining expertise in all features of infertility treatment, Dr Bajaj is adept at treating infertility in both women as well as men. Owing to her higher education and fine skills, she dexterously handles complex issues which are usually taken care of by 'infertility experts' and board-certified regenerative endocrinologists who have finished their training in obstetrics and gynaecology. Giving best counseling and also the best required treatment to the couples as they want to know the issue in a transparent manner, Dr Bajaj provides various treatments like IVF, Intra-cytoplasmic sperm injection (ICSI), embryo transfer, Surgical Sperm retrieval techniques and others. Desperately craving for having their own baby, aspiring parents are offered positive prospects and perfect counseling by Dr Bajaj, who works with the motive of spreading cheers of parental bliss and is highly skilled to do so.

Nurture - The Abode Of Euphoria

Under the exemplary leadership of Dr Bajaj, The Nurture IVF Clinic at Naraina Vihar, New Delhi, is consistently striving to offer the best solutions to couples seeking treatment of infertility, since its very origin, and is equipped with high end technology and up-to-date infrastructure to provide one of the best fertility treatments such as IVF, Surrogacy, ICSI, and IUI procedures. Conforming to the international standards with regard to its techniques and procedures, the Clinic has a team of accomplished IVF Specialists, Embryologists,

Gynaecologists and Endoscopists. With an outstanding success rate, The Nurture IVF Clinic is the best in Delhi and is one of the top fertility clinics in India.

Focused on helping couples to sail out from trauma of infertility by providing them appropriate and cost-effective treatments to have their own baby, The Nurture IVF Clinic offers a plethora of services such as IVF, ICSI, IUI, Egg Donation, Embryo Donation, Assisted Hatching, Surrogacy, Embryo Freezing, Male Infertility Services, Sperm Banks and other Natural Infertility Treatments. In addition, it also provides infertility books, infertility support and drugs with encouraging emotional and moral support.

As one of the forerunners in the techniques of ICSI and having done more than 2000 cycles with success rates of around 25% – 30%, The Nurture IVF Clinic is the first unit in India to initiate the technique of Assisted Laser Hatching – a boon for elderly patients or those with the history of repeated failures – as it improves their chances of pregnancy. Being one of the oldest infertility clinics in Delhi, offering one of the most advanced and internationally competitive ART programs and services, The Nurture IVF center is equipped with the state-of-the-art 'Embryology Laboratory' and the staff comprises highly trained professionals. With an undeterred mission of offering fertility-related medical attention, emotional advice, ethical values, and state-of-the-art technical support to couples who are going through hard times due to their inability to conceive a child. Propelled by the motivating force which Dr Bajaj emanates, the team at The Nurture IVF centre, strives to provide the best medical services at par with the international standards at cost-effective price. As the director of the clinic and leader of eminent group of IVF specialist doctors, she not only shares her valuable experience but inspires them to produce the best result for each and every patient.

Thriving Under A Rich Legacy

Being brought up in an army background, owing to her father being a reputed gynaecologist in the army, discipline has always been the guiding principle of her life. Her refined character is a fruitful outcome of the cantonment milieu enveloping her formative years. Inspired by a gynaecologist father and an anesthesiologist mother, Dr Bajaj chose to excel in the medical profession alike her parents. They sowed in her the vital seeds of morality, which has enabled her to climb the escalator of success while simultaneously being an epitome of trust, faith and compassion for her patients.

Gentleness Personified

Being a very soft-spoken lady with a friendly demeanor, Dr Bajaj is a kind-hearted personality who is ever ready to help her patients at any hour of the day and even night. Eminently renowned and widely popular for imparting miraculous results in the field of Assisted Reproductive Technology, she has been a popular face on various TV channels, Magazines and journals contributing her valuable insights to the common people as an act of altruism.

Incessant Strive To Success

According to Dr Bajaj, the motto behind laying the very foundation of The Nurture IVF Clinic is to add a spark of hope to the gloomy lives of childless couples. Not leaving any stone unturned to give the best, she dexterously plays the part of not only a doctor, but of a mentor as well and is capable of playing many roles in a great manner at the same time. Bent on making the treatment beneficial for the patients, she is on a never ending quest to update herself with the latest developments and technology in the field of ART. No wonder, she has numerous satisfied patients who thank her wholeheartedly as they don the new roles of parents.

As a proficient scholar, Dr Bajaj has received the coveted National Science Talent Award by the government of India (1986-1991). She also won the Best Resident and Post graduate Award in Obstetrics and Gynaecology from Sir Ganga Ram Hospital, New Delhi, in 2001. However, she vehemently believes that the real award is the exhilaration which she is able to bring to the childless couples and their families as she hands over their bundles of joy to them.

Chapter 9

Moral Issues: Always Upfront

Dr Archana Dhawan Bajaj is strictly a 'by- the- rules' IVF specialist and her scruples always come first in her vocation. As is her wont, Dr (Mrs) Bajaj is never shy of scrutiny and speaking from the front against anything unethical or unwarranted. She is never reticent when any cause celebre in the domain presented itself and speaks her mind without hedging her bets. She would not mince words or try to sound worldly wise. She is a straight shooter so far as ethicality of the vocation is concerned.

The issue of no-nonsense magazine **Outlook** March 14, 2022: **Salute to the women in Leadership** bears witness to how Dr (Mrs) Bajaj is reckoned. Dr (Mrs) Bajaj built her reputation as a woman leader of substance through her unvarnished views on issues confronting her domain. Thanks to her views loud and clear on issues of propriety, Dr Archana made the grade of Union Finance Minister Nirmala Sitaraman, Nita Ambani, Mandhira Kapoor, Meenal Goswamy, Soma Mondal, Chandni Kapadia, Deepika Padukone, Meghna Ghai Puri, Sohini Sastri, Dr Nirmala

Pandey, Shilpa Kulshreshtha, Rochita Venkataraman, Ranjoo Mann, Neha Rastogi, Alpa Kapadia Teli, Harnaaz Kaur Sandhu and Shalya Raj when the prestigious magazine aggregated its pick of woman leaders worthy of salute. Her interview in this Outlook issue is presented here without filter. In the interview, she earned the nickname of White Stork in the lives of Couples, White Stork is supposed to be bringer of new born babies.

Long before regulation rules were put in place not long ago, she was firmly for the regulation of IVF industry which, according to her, was going haywire in absence of it. Being a stickler for fair practices, Dr Bajaj always asked for regulation albeit good one, from the front as her centre Nurture has no underbelly. She always felt ignominy was being heaped upon a sacrosanct procedure due to unbridled unscrupulous players in the domain. She earnestly wanted them to be banished to save fair practitioners from the blot. She held a well thought out regulation rules were in favour of real and credible fertility experts and their centres.

Dr Bajaj felt concerned that wannabe IVF experts had mushroomed to tap into the desperation of burgeoning infertile couples and instead of perfecting procedure, these shady centres had perfected the art of duping unsuspecting childless couples. Whenever something unbecoming came into open about IVF practice, she would lose no time to express her moral indignation loud and clear.

Here are samples of her positions she took on different issues when the crunch came-

On onus of infertility being thrust upon women-

She always resented the fact that when it came to infertility, women would invariably be ticked off. This skewed thinking is now slowly giving way to fair assessment involving women and men but it took ivf experts like Dr (Mrs) Bajaj to express strong views against this ill-founded stereotype. She always held that women are more sinned against than sinning when it came to infertility. It took long but Dr (Mrs) Bajaj and her ilk finally made men out of closet to share the onus of infertility in case they, instead of their wives, contributed to the condition.

By a rough estimate about 30 percent infertility in India is thanks to men. So, it is prejudicial to attribute sterility on fair sexes alone. Men must come upfront to take the onus. Infertility in India has become quite pervasive in men these days. Acquiescing it early and going for test early in fact spare women a lot of hassles and result into getting treated and having child early. Until not long ago, male infertility was largely an ignored phenomenon in India and women were subjected to a lot of social stigmas for being unable to bear children despite being in fine fettle for fertility. Though situation has improved a lot but there is still need to hammer home the point so that the fact percolates down to all and sundry that men's deficiency too are causing childlessness. Sooner men realised this better for making a family.

Dr (Mrs) Bajaj says equal importance must be assigned to male infertility in course of quest for bundles of joy. More awareness is needed to sink in this fact of fertility. Early testing of men is advisable. It should now be taken as official that infertility is not just a woman's problem and it is important to raise awareness about male infertility and the causative factors. In men, the most common reasons for infertility include a low sperm count and poor motility of the sperm. Other factors such as male infertility are excessive consumption of foods that increase estrogens in the blood, long-term inhalation of toxins in the air, erectile dysfunction, early ejaculation of semen, cancer or infection of the genital system and diabetes also contribute to the condition.'

Dr (Mrs) Bajaj further says, 'Men usually put off testing to avoid embarrassment. However, getting diagnosed at an early stage will not only save discomfort and expense but also help in timely treatment. The bright side is that recent medical breakthroughs have helped even men with very few sperms to become fathers. It is also important to make certain lifestyle changes such as quitting smoking and drinking, and consuming a healthy diet, all of which can help in preventing infertility and avoiding any possible complications'

Infertility, both in men and women, is on the rise in India. As per estimates, there has been a 20% to 30% rise in infertility in the country in the last five years. Infertility is broadly used to denote a range of conditions, which affect both men and women.

According to Dr (Mrs) Bajaj some treatment options for addressing male infertility include the following.

- ***Intrauterine Insemination (IUI)*** –This method can be tried when the sperm count is at least 10 million. In this process, the semen is washed using special methods in a lab and a small quantity of sperms are placed, using a thin tube, inside the woman's womb. This is a simple, inexpensive procedure.

- ***Intracytoplasmic Sperm Injection (ICSI)*** – This is akin to a test-tube baby procedure. Eggs from the women are removed with a needle under sonography control and placed under a microscope. Each sperm is picked up with a needle and injected directly into the egg with a micromanipulator. The eggs then fertilize and divide. After two to three days, the embryo is placed in the womb.

- ***PESA, TESA***– At times even when a hormone test is normal, there may be no sperms in the semen. In such cases, the sperms can be removed directly from the testes using a tiny needle. These are then injected into the egg using the ICSI procedure.

- ***Donor sperms***– There are also cases of complete testicular failure with abnormal hormones and no sperms. In such cases, donor sperms obtained from a semen bank. This is then injected into the woman.

On IVF being misused for children in much advanced age

When such news as 70- or 75-year-old women getting baby with the help of IVF surfaced, Dr (Mrs) lost no time to bat for capping the age limit of going for ivf. She said, 'yes of course advancement in IVF has made age of women irrelevant. But that does not mean that we should lose all sense of proportion and prosperity. No woman should be encouraged to become a mother at such an advanced age. The ideal cut off age for IVF is 47- 50 but if the woman is extremely fit the age limit can be maximised to 52-53 years. To use ivf on a woman aged over 60 or seventy is clearly a misuse of the technology. The issue of upbringing of the babies seeing the light of the day must not be lost sight of.'

On Single parenting-

When Karan Johar, the famous 'no holds barred' Bollywood Director flaunted his twin **Ruhee and Yash** using surrogacy, Dr (Mrs) Bajaj was quick to express her moral indignation. Without mincing words, she dubbed this act cavalier and a slur on the sacrosanct.

Karan Johar's act in fact had jolted almost entire fertility expert's fraternity. Karan Johar was in 'gay abandon' on becoming a single parent to twins through surrogacy. He and his cohorts in the Bollywood went gaga over this acquisition but fertility experts, by and large, expressed anguish dubbing this as his indiscretion in the name of individual freedom. To use his bug bear Kangana Ranaut's portrayal, the Movie mafia and snooty Johar had muddied the sacrosanct surrogacy (as depicted by its practitioners) instead of being its flag bearer. They had said, 'Karan Johar becoming single dad of twins, Ruhee and Yash, has perhaps hastened the ban on commercial surrogacy (renting a womb) in India. Audacity of Karan Johar proved last hurrah for surrogacy.'

Especially, Dr. (Mrs) Bajaj was perturbed by Johor's indiscretion. Dr. Bajaj, well known for practising only ethical surrogacy, had said, 'I am totally against single parenthood and never entertained anyone for this in Nurture. Karan Johar has brought ignominy on otherwise a sacrosanct process that empowers poor surrogates and hands bundles of joys to hapless childless couples. Being single and because of what Johar is perceived to be, he is not at all competent to provide ideal setting and family environment for the upbringing of two unsuspecting babies.'

Hot on the heels of Johar's announcement of having child 'trophies', Supreme Court had to intervene to compel central government to give undertaking that henceforth single parenting would not be allowed. Only infertile married Indian couples would be entitled to take the route. Had the Assisted Reproductive (ART) Regulation Bill been in place at that time, Karan Johar would not have been able to fulfil his wish of having bundles of joy.

Dr. Bajaj had said, 'Acts like that of Johar and his likes have been the cause of disrepute of this sacrosanct contract for co-operation in fertility and sharing of joys of birth of a baby. IVF and surrogacy have helped many childless couples but trend towards single parenthood can have far reaching effect on child's behaviour and impact several areas of life, including emotional, mental growth and social behaviours of the child.'

On 10-year-old pregnant rape survivor

Dr (Mrs) Bajaj's heart bled for a 10-year-old pregnant rape survivor. She had demanded her immediate deliverance from agony of foetus. She had said the case was beyond all bearing for her. Her heart ached for the hapless girl.

In 2017, the rape survivor of Chandigarh, had approached the Supreme Court, seeking permission to abort her 26-week-old foetus, plaintively pleading that her pelvis was unable to hold the baby. Regardless of apex court's ruling, Gynaecologists across the country wanted her free from foetus forthwith. She was allegedly raped by her uncle.

Expressing outrage and anguish, obstetricians, gynaecologists and assisted birthing experts across the board had empathised with girl's misery. They demanded in unison that she must immediately be rescued from the fatal foetus.

This painful cause celebre had jolted the collective consciousness of the nation no end. Obstetricians, gynaecologists and IVF experts reacted with utmost indignation going way beyond the legal and health risk issues involved in this.

The girl was really in a terrible predicament and needed immediate deliverance from the foetus wedged into her. Nothing could be more loathsome than the scenario in which an innocent girl had been shoved into.

Dr. (Mrs) Bajaj was visibly upset at the plight of the unfortunate girl. Shehad said, 'It's heart-wrenching indeed, seeing such young girls getting pregnant. We as birthing professionals are primed to see mature ladies bearing pain with fortitude and not to be jolted by it but this 10-year-old girl's misery has breached our pain threshold. I am feeling the prick in my conscience.'

Dr (Mrs) Bajaj had added, 'A girl of 10 getting pregnant itself is a threat to life and a trauma hard to bear. It becomes worse if she is bearing a foetus due to rape; the trauma goes beyond all bearing.'

She had added, 'Talking only physically, the greatest danger is to the pelvic floor. Girls may start ovulating and menstruating as early as age 8 these days, though the average is around 12 to 13. The younger they are, more the traumas would be. Once menstruation starts, growth tends to slow in girls. The pelvic floor isn't developed enough yet. And even if puberty onset is happening earlier, pelvises are not maturing any faster. Her life is for sure at higher risk and results might be more often than not horrific. Girls may labour for days; many of them die. The babies they bear often don't survive labour either.'

Heralding the White Stork in Lives of Couples!

As pioneering IVF specialist of India, Dr. Archana Dhawan Bajaj, Medical Director and IVF Doctor at The Nurture IVF Centre, has brought happiness in the lives of thousands of couples in her career of two decades. The recipient of several honours and awards for her stellar contribution to the relatively young speciality, was inspired by her father, an army personnel. On International Women's Day, she shares her happening life with the Outlook.

What perceptible difference do you see in people today as compared to when you started the speciality?

When we look back at our journey of last 15-20 years, when we started The NURTURE IVF Centre, it was fraught with challenges. ICF was an emerging speciality and not much heard or known about by the public. It not only included convincing couples with fertility issues to go for it, but most importantly to convince the male partner and their participation in the treatment because of the huge obstacle-The Male ego! The societal mind set was such that women were blamed for in case of infertility problems. Add to it limited public information on about IVF treatment. We have come a long way since then. Today, couples and people in general are more accepting and it is not a taboo subject anymore, especially in the urban population. Men are the surprise package who have a more liberal outlook!

Counselling is integral for the IVF treatment to be effective. How does it help?

Yes, counselling is a very integral part of the IVF treatment like any other. Nevertheless, the doctor's words in our speciality carries much more weightage because the completion of a family is at stake and couple comes to us as a last resort. Unlike in other parts of the country, there is a marked difference in the way the IVF speciality is looked at in the north. In the north, the reproductive treatment is more doctor specific where couples prefer going to the speciality rather than going to counsellors at corporate-like clinics that have mushroomed in the last couple of years. Though counsellors are good at their work, but when it comes to couples making the choices, it's always the doctors advise that is final.

What are the issues that really traumatise women opting for IVF treatment?

The fact that they are not getting pregnant is the foremost of their concerns. Family and social pressures are the other concerns that rankles their emotional and mental frame of mind. The other biggest concern is the affordability of the treatment because it's a long-drawn process and this also plays on their mind. Also, as a clinician, I can handhold them through the best customised treatment for the best results, but then the outcome is not in our hands, which again is a stress that they have to cope with in the event of a failure and cost implications involved. This shatters the confidence of women because they can't face failure and sink into depression.

Advancement of medicine and procedures are giving better results. What is the latest in IVF?

A lot of changes and developments have occurred in IVF and fertility speciality, particularly in the last ten years, with frozen cycles being one of them. Blastocyst Culture, Embryo Cryo Preservation, Assisted Hatching, Polscope Microscope, Pre-Implantation and Genetic Diagnosis PGD are among some other treatments for which Nurture Centre is known for.

What is the reason for increasing infertility in the society?

There are multiple reasons, lifestyle being one of the major contributors. Smoking, alcohol, recreational indulgence, couples with different working hours, too much of travel and stress, environmental factors and exposure to different kinds of bacterial and viral disease such as the Covid -19 have only aggravated the reproductive ability of women.

What would you like to share with women based on your experience of life?

Learn to give back to the society what you have earned from it. And give the best of your best in whatever you do, because there are no shortcuts to success. Also, women as compared to men are emotionally stronger and give selflessly. Women are powerful, keep it up!

Chapter - 10

Womb Wise

This chapter is 'pregnant' with wisdom about fertility, aggregated from Dr (Mrs) Bajaj and other credible sources. These words, if read in earnest can make quest of bundle of joys a walk in the park. The chapter should pave the way for a successful pregnancy through IVF. It will serve as a bellwether for motherhood seekers.

The sage advice for IVF to be sure successful is that there is not much time to lose. Time being of essence, there is a ripe time for fast forward to IVF. If a couple seeking to make family follows timelines and is wombly wise advice of a credible fertility expert, there is no reason that quest for bundle of joy should end in disappointment.

The timeline is paramount in seeking pregnancy and then taking home a baby to fill one's life with joy. Keeping in mind the guidelines about calendar of fecundity set by a reliable birthing expert makes the quest a lot easier. There are tipping points in birthing journey that must be kept in mind. Loss of time means odds of having bundle of joys starting to diminish.

Infertility can be extremely distressing. For many, it can be an isolating and incredibly painful experience. Dreams seem shattered and expectations divided between two poles. Negativity prevails and there seem no light at the end of the tunnel. One should shake off such feelings forthwith and consult one of the best infertility specialists and try to figure out the possible solution to get out of this situation and attain pregnancy.

The problem is that most of the male and female affected with infertility condition are not aware of when to consult the infertility doctor. As a result, the problem gets bigger and bigger and reaches to the point of mental, physical and emotional distress and agony. Being abreast of when is the right time to consult an IVF specialist helps pregnancy seekers avoid the extreme infertility complication and condition.

Conditions and time that puts pregnancy seekers on notice regarding exigency of seeing a fertility expert.

1. When things do not pan out accordingly

You are a married couple and trying to conceive longer than you ever thought possible. You are confused about why it does not yield any conception. At this juncture, you should seek medical help immediately. Immediately does not mean that the situation is grave, it means you should not let the condition to deteriorate further so much so that it reaches to the point of extreme complication.

2. It is taking more time than expected

Sometimes we take things for granted and only wake up when things start moving away from us. As a couple, if you are not able to produce reproduction even after a long time and several efforts to achieve conception, get in mind that it is the time to move to a reputed IVF expert to get your infertility condition thoroughly analysed. Intended or unintended delay, both will push your existing infertility issue to the next level where you might have had to go through an extreme ordeal to achieve pregnancy and deliver a child.

3. It is more than one year, you are still trying

Even if you are young enough to wait for so many years to get things aligned according to your expectation, it is widely recommended that you should seek medical help when it is more than a year of the unsuccessful chase of getting pregnant naturally. In other words, if a male and female involved in a timely performed sexual intercourse for more than a year and did not achieve conception, no matter what they must consult the best infertility specialist and discuss their issue with him/ her.

4. When the age of the woman is 35 or above

Infertility or fail to achieve pregnancy has a direct relationship with the age of the women. After the age of 35 or above, the chances of achieving pregnancy dwindle abruptly. Moreover, the chances of miscarriage also go up drastically. Hence, you do not get pregnant within the six months of unprotected sexual practices; you should knock the door of an infertility specialist and discuss your problem.

Must Keep time in Your sights

Keeping track of time is the best way to go about attaining pregnancy. Sample the example- Supposing one is around 25 and has been trying for a baby for a year but yet unable to conceive, then the woman is question must see a fertility expert. If she is in 30s, should try six months window before consulting her fertility specialist. But if you are over 35, you have no time to stand and stare; consult your specialist immediately. Infertility or fail to achieve pregnancy has a direct relationship with the age of the women. After the age of 35 or above, the chances of achieving pregnancy dwindle abruptly. With age eggs in a woman gradually decrease. Moreover, the chances of miscarriage also go up drastically. Hence, you do not get pregnant within the six months of unprotected sexual practices; you should knock the door of an infertility specialist and discuss your problem.

Reckon with AMH (Anti-Mullerian Hormone) level

AMH is a crucial aspect in prospect of conception. Its test is used to a woman's ability to produce eggs that can be fertilized. This test is critical in assessing ovarian reserve. If this reserve is high, there may be better chance of getting pregnant. A woman's ovaries can make thousands of eggs during child bearing years. The number declines as woman gets older. AMH test could be potent pointer to prospect of conception.

Fertility via DINK- a dire strait

Double Income No Kids (DINK) trend is putting fertility at back burner-

This seemingly bizarre trend is the harsh reality of present-day quest for motherhood. The temptation for big money & high society life is in fact spoiling urge for parenthood. As lure of lucre is becoming be all and end all of a conjugal life, urge for motherhood among career women is at its lowest ebb. In the hot career pursuit, a large number of people all over the country including in Delhi are attaining the age when parenthood becomes difficult as they lose their fecundity.

DINK couples delay and put the idea of having bundle of joy on the back burner till they amass lot of wealth and wherewithal to indulge in high life. They are part of the popular culture, infiltrating to India from West that puts carnal pleasures and joys of sex far above the happiness of motherhood. A growing number of career women are being found visiting assisted fertility clinics in India in their late thirties and forties.

Though some Hollywood heroines sporadically flaunt their baby bumps, as if celebrating motherhood with élan but the urge for parenthood in high society where they come from, is now only skin deep.

The growth of the DINK is reflecting the lives of thousands of those couples who choose to be childless in pursuit of their career ambitions. A shallow lifestyle embodied by DINK adds nothing to the propagation of the race and family line. Hence, they are contributing towards a major decline of the civilization that has set in.

Though it is a common phenomenon in the West, a developing country India too has been prejudiced by the DINK's trend. There are varied reasons why some married couples in metropolises choose not to have children.

Inclination towards the ongoing transformation of the socio-economic context and expanded work opportunities have hugely lured talented women who are ready to compete with men to make a move from home to the office. In the process, many choose careers or one-time motherhood and love the work challenge or resort to delayed marriage prospects.

Dr (Mrs) Bajaj says, 'Throughout their lives these couples prioritize their work for a family life and plan to settle down for a family life when they near the age of 30-32 (when they achieve much in life and are financially firm). They hardly realize that women have lower pregnancy chances after 30. The fertility of a woman starts declining after a she crosses 27. Men's fertility too starts dropping after 35. The chances of miscarriage, ectopic pregnancy or chromosomal abnormality go up as you come of age. Hence it is always recommendable for couples to plan for a baby when they are in their twenties.' The peak fertility occurs between 20-30, then starts declining by 20% after 30, 50% after 35 and 95% after 50'. Consequent to the declining rates of fertility after 30 and high-risk pregnancy after this age; many couples end up with no kids at all.

Kids or Career? Career couples galore are today pitted against this dilemma. Thanks to constant advancement in IVF, this twain can very well meet. IVF has answer to this impasse. You cannot fault couples of today seeking best of both the worlds. In absence of IVF, the choice between urge for motherhood and career would have been a tight rope walking. Gratefully, IVF gives a long rope. Thanks to this hope technology, there is always light at end of the long tunnel.

Temptation for bundle of money before having bundle of joy is the dilemma that couples of today generally confront. It is not to say that their lure for amassing wealth and high society life are diminishing their fondness for kids. Only that they want to provide well for their offspring and high society life. In the scheme of things of new age marital life, postponing of making family is not entirely a senseless idea. Of course, trend of planning making of family quite late is catching up in the new age marital life of India.

IVF is rightly being called as hope technology of assisted birthing. The continued advancement in this technology is zeroing in all the problems being faced by couples in modern context. Freezing of eggs for later use in attaining motherhood after settling question of career is catching up in India too. Couples don't have to remain childless if they don't wish to. Gone are the days when couples had to choose between having kids or focusing on their careers and pleasures.

Men's fertility in India may be imperilled by Hepatitis B

Hepatitis does not endanger liver alone; it is a recipe for infertility in men too. If, as stats go, 52 million people in India live with hepatitis virus, men in million might be in danger of losing their fecundity. But there is little awareness about Hepatitis B's collateral damage on fertility. Of the five hepatitis viruses, hepatitis B is associated with impaired fertility.

Studies have indicated that those with HB are 1.59 times more likely to experience infertility than individuals who are not infected. Hepatitis B virus' S protein is known to lower sperm motility and reduce the fertilization rate of sperms by more than half. Hepatitis B and C viruses can be transmitted from the mother to baby, via sexual contact or upon contact with infected blood.

Hepatitis does not have any effect on the normal functioning of the ovarian or uterine glands. However, this virus impacts spermatogenesis negatively in males. This causes a reduction in the sperm count, free testosterone levels, motility, viability, and morphology which further impacts overall fertility and ability to produce an offspring in them.

It is imperative to counsel couples who have been tested positive for hepatitis and seeking fertility treatment. This would in turn enable them to understand the transmission risk of the disease. Any assisted reproduction techniques should be suggested only once proper treatment is done and the viral load is reduced.

Transmission risk from mother to baby increases by 80% to 90% in Hepatitis B cases and 11% in Hepatitis C positive cases, where there is high viral load. Some ways to reduce this risk include semen washing, administering the uninfected partner with hepatitis B vaccination, and treatment with Interferon and Ribavirin. Many couples would have doubts, fears, and misconceptions in their mind about this condition. It is important to encourage couples to come out and talk about these fears and apprehensions through support and peer groups as in the West. These can help them make empowered choices about safe, effective avenues to explore vis-à-vis the critical decision of expanding their families.

Sexual & Reproductive Illiteracy leads to Fertility Disorders in India

Utter lack of awareness about sexual and reproductive health can lead to a litany of sexual disorders. Illiteracy among adolescents and youth in India regarding these matters may put them in jeopardy. Fertility is the major casualty.

Sample this: only 26% of adolescent girls know that a condom should be used only once, and only 34% understood that oral contraceptive pills must be taken daily

Of all the important consequences of poor sexual health is infertility. This is because not maintaining sexual health can lead to various diseases such as STDs which may eventually contribute to loss of fertility. Both men and women should aim at maintaining their sexual and reproductive health by highlighting any specific or unknown symptoms, and address concerns at the earliest. This includes undergoing regular check-ups at various stages of their life.

Sexual health refers to avoiding infections and illnesses, and taking responsibility to ensure that we protect ourselves and others, emotionally and physically. It is integral to a person's overall health. Lack of awareness can lead to a person being unable to understand the underlying causes of sexual disorders and seek appropriate help. One of the greatest barriers to the WHO's vision of sexual health and promoting responsible sexual behaviour is the unwillingness of individuals to discuss their sexual problems. It is important to create awareness on the fact that sexual health issues must be addressed in a timely manner. This can be done by talking about it with a health care provider and your partner.'

Surveys and studies suggest that Indian adolescents and youth do not receive relevant information on sexual matters from reliable sources. There is an overall lack of awareness about sexual and reproductive health in men as well as in women alike in India, which may cause them to suffer a number of disorders. Sexual health refers to the many factors that impact sexual function and reproduction. These include a variety of physical, mental and emotional factors. Disorders that affect any of these factors can impact a person's physical and emotional health, as well as his or her relationships and self-image.

Some examples of reproductive system disorders include cancers of the cervix or prostate gland, infertility issues, gynaecological problems such as endometriosis, urinary system problems, STDs, sexual dysfunction, painful intercourse, concerns regarding "normal" or acceptable sexual behaviour and lifestyles, and birth control.

Tips to ensure maintenance of good sexual health.

- Eat healthy. Healthy food nourishes the body and allows it to be at its best in many situations, including sex.

- Avoid smoking. Smoking reduces your vitality. Tobacco also leads to constriction of blood vessels including in the genitals. In men, this reduction in the blood flow can lead to difficulty in having or maintaining an erection. In women, it can cause lubrication reduction.

- Maintain a healthy weight. Overweight or obese people are at a greater risk of hypertension, hypercholesterolemia and diabetes, medical conditions that may be detrimental to a good sexual health.

- Limit alcohol consumption. Consuming large quantities of alcohol can have a negative impact on men and women's sexual capacities.

- Communicate with your partner. Feel comfortable with your partner and talk to them about anything that may be worrying you.

- Protect yourself. Safety is always first. Using a condom reduces the risks of both an unwanted pregnancy and contracting a sexually transmitted infection (STI).

A pregnant Mother risks her heart for the bundle of joy

A pregnant mother also carries risk of heart disease in her womb. **Monitoring BP during pregnancy can avert the hazard of heart disease later**

Pregnancy induces hypertension in the mother which used to be viewed as normal. But not anymore. Recent research has shown that women with high blood pressure during pregnancy stand at a greater risk of developing heart diseases later in life. It can lead to still birth too.

So, hypertension is a crucial aspect of the motherhood. If blood pressure is monitored and necessary intervention is done, other complications like seizures and still birth can well be averted.

As per recent statistics, about 7% to 10% of pregnant women experience pregnancy induced hypertension (PIH). This is a condition in which a woman's blood pressure rises way above the normal levels. PIH is a temporary condition in most women. However, in others it can continue post-delivery as well and left untreated, can lead to preeclampsia.

A woman needs to do much more than watching her weight and taking vitamins during pregnancy. There is also a need to carefully monitor vitals especially the blood pressure levels. This is all the more necessary for women who have an existing history of high blood pressure, kidney ailments, diabetes, history of preeclampsia during first pregnancy, or those pregnant with multiple fetuses.

PIH develops a resistance in the blood vessels, affecting the blood flow throughout the body. This includes the blood flow to the placenta and uterus, which can cause growth problems for the unborn baby. PIH can also lead to premature detachment of the placenta from the uterus and thereby stillbirth. An increased blood pressure means the heart must work harder to pump blood. This, in later life, can cause seizures and heart diseases in such women and in rare cases can also become fatal.

It is imperative to monitor fluctuations in BP during pregnancy since not all of it can be attributed to PIH. Post-delivery, the BP levels should be monitored through ABPM (ambulatory blood pressure monitoring) regularly.'

Poor menstrual hygiene may be recipe for infertility

Poor menstrual hygiene poses serious health risks, like reproductive and urinary tract infections which can result in future infertility and birth complications. More Awareness on Menstrual hygiene & Management needed in India

Statistics indicate that India has over 355 million menstruating women and girls, but many of them face uncomfortable and undignified experience with menstrual hygiene management. Despite national and international level push to address this issue through various social media platforms, campaigns, availability of eco-friendly or biodegradable menstrual products, etc., there is still ambiguity around the issue especially in the rural areas. There is a need to raise awareness on these aspects especially among rural school going girls.

Informed choice is an important aspect of women's reproductive and sexual health. This is also important with regard to menstrual hygiene wherein they have access to information about the products available, their advantages and how to use and dispose them, and the freedom to choose a product depending on their needs, and the socio-economic contexts in which they live in.

Despite progressive statistics, menstrual hygiene is an essential aspect of female health which is grossly neglected in India. Although there are several government initiatives which have brought significant improvement in the number of women having access to sanitary pads, many in the rural areas continue using unhygienic alternatives. Awareness needs to be raised not only on maintaining hygiene, but also on the availability of sustainable alternatives such as biodegradable sanitary pads and menstrual cups. They are beneficial to both women's health and the environment.

Period talk is an extremely important aspect of sexual education in young girls. It must be imparted at the right age and time leading up to menarche. There is a need to make them aware that inadequate attention to menstrual hygiene can lead to many infections and even cervical cancer over time. Awareness is needed not only among the girls but also their mothers and family on how important it is to offer support and understanding during this critical phase.

Lack of menstrual hygiene after the birth of a baby can also impact the mother's health leading to issues such as urinary tract infection (UTI) and reproductive tract infections (RTIs). Awareness on the use of hygienic methods and proper disposal of waste is a must.

There is a strong need for creating awareness among women of hygienic practices during the menstrual, partum and postpartum periods. Unclean practices can increase the risk of infections in new mothers impacting their health.

Thus, apart from using proper sanitary products, it is also imperative to ensure that they wash their intimate area well, change pads from as and when required, among other things.

As a society, the stigma around periods or menstruation must be overcome. it is imperative to understand that there is nothing shameful or impure about and that women have the right to access to sanitation and good menstrual hygiene. Building knowledge and support are key as is dispelling myths and taboos surrounding menstruation by talking about it proactively without shame

Count Chromosomes while Pregnant to avert Child with Down Syndrome

Despite all kinds of loving and brave words about Down Syndrome ones, the last thing that a mother to be would wish is a genetically abnormal child. 'Friends may not count chromosomes' but it is most advisable that a pregnant mother should count them lest they harbour a baby with extra 21st chromosome that leads to Down Syndrome. Non- invasive and a blood-based latest test is now available.

Down Syndrome is a condition in which a child is born with an extra 21st chromosome. Down syndrome is a critical gene defect found at a rate of one in two thousand babies born to women below the age of 35 years and one in 50 above 35 years of age. Many genetic abnormalities including chromosomal abnormalities such as Down Syndrome can be detected with genetic testing during pregnancy.

Genetic disorders constitute an increasing proportion of stillbirths, child mortality, morbidity, disability, and Down Syndrome. For a better outcome of pregnancy, women need to be cautious about some genetic defects and those can be either due to single-gene mutations and chromosomal abnormalities. Expectant women now do not need to worry. Next-generation sequencing technology (NGS) has all potential to transform the ways experts deal with genetic defects to ensure a better outcome of pregnancy.

Other disorders that can and should be detected include Cystic fibrosis, Muscular dystrophy, Hemophilia, Polycystic kidney disease, Sickle cell disease, and Thalassemia.

The fear that engulfs every expectant parent these days, is the outcome of pregnancy: whether the baby will be healthy or have any defects, unfortunately, if the genetic problem is detected late, then it would lead to the birth of a physically and/or cognitively challenged child.

The standard method where one can do a genetic screening of the pregnant woman either in the 1st 3 months or next three months of pregnancy. In the first three months, traditionally you can do the dual marker blood test in combination with the sonography examination of the baby's nuchal thickness at 11 weeks. However, nowadays instead of doing a Dual Marker Blood test, one can do a Non-Invasive Prenatal Test (NIPT) on the blood of the mother from 10th (2.5-months) to 20th (5-months) weeks of pregnancy.

Down's syndrome can be screened in the second trimester by doing a screening on the mother's blood called the

Quadruple Marker Test in association with the ultrasound examination of the baby at 18 weeks of pregnancy. One can also do a NIPT test on a mother's blood. If the Dual Marker, NT scan, Quadruple Marker, NIPT comes positive then confirmation of Down Syndrome is done by doing the genetic testing by karyotype method on the tissue obtained by chorion villus sampling or amniocentesis.

NGS technologies including NIPT are ahead of all other technologies as they provide high-quality genetic information with accuracy. The next-generation sequencing is designed to employ massively parallel strategies to produce large amounts of DNA sequencing, from multiple samples at very high-throughput and at a high degree of sequence coverage. NGS also is more effective in assessing mosaicism in embryos, following PGT.

With genetic defects being a big issue in newborn babies, a host of screening tests are employed to map this. After the various screening, we come to know the root cause, and then treatment is done. These are some very critical tests to be performed at different stages of pregnancy to detect foetal abnormalities.

Chapter- 11

Of Baby & Bath Water

Commercial surrogacy has strangely been declared guilty despite being found innocent, ignoring the dictum of natural justice- innocent until proved guilty. It was banned on the basis of flimsy and fanciful allegation that poor women who rented wombs were being exploited. Oddly enough, not a single surrogate mother turned up to allege exploitation.

By a law in parliament named Surrogacy (Regulation) Bill 2020 in 2021, the lives- transforming sacrosanct cooperative birthing was banned in the name of regulating two decades of booming practice in India to the chagrin of fertility experts. All arguments of fertility experts fell flat on deaf ears.

It was win- win practice indeed- childless couples who had no hope of having children got ones and on the other hand, poor women who rented their wombs got new life- two life transforming births in a manner of speaking. Poor women whose lives were transformed could hardly make both ends meet.

Surrogacy had been a significant part of Dr Archana Dhawan's bumper IVF baby yield. And she has been a witness to this process greatly empowering poor women who rented their wombs for the childless couples on the brink of losing hope of bundles of joy for want of wombs to hold the embryos and nurture them. The rented wombs that housed happiness for mothers bereft of uterus were leap of faith for many a childless couple. Surrogacy in Nurture has been a saga of sacrosanct contracts for bundles of joy.

The ban on commercial surrogacy in India has left Dr Archana Dhawan Bajaj baffled wondering as to what led to this arbitrary step. Nurture stands witness that the allegation and perception that surrogate mothers were exploited was ill founded. She did not grudge regulation but banning it altogether, she thinks, is like throwing out the baby with the bath water. As Dr Archana is a law-abiding fertility expert, commercial surrogacy is out of bound for Nurture now but she still feels a tug at heart at the cessation of this innocuous process and for the loss of those women who were at the receiving end.

An apologist of well-regulated surrogacy, Dr Bajaj feels that the ban is the outcome of excessive zeal of reform. How fervently she wishes the sacrosanct process of cooperative motherhood is restored! When the ban was being formalised, she even argued for utmost regulation in place to save the contract of hope. She has many stories to tell how renting of wombs transformed the lives of many a poor woman who looked at the opportunity as godsend.

As need of surrogacy increases by the day due to different unavoidable factors, Dr Bajaj feels that had fair commercial surrogacy continued, India would have become the greatest exporter of joy to global women resulting into massive influx of foreign exchange to the country into the bargain. While doing surrogacy, Dr Bajaj acted as keeper of faith for poor women who rented their wombs when allowed and still has bonding with them.

Booming 'rent a womb' bliss and biz was demolished in one fell swoop by the law which though is in place with good intention but unreasonable and misplaced. Anand in Gujarat, which also translates as bundle of joy, once being surrogacy hub, the happy confluence of Mother and Milk, it was looked at as cooperative fertility just as cooperative milk. Surrogacy was reckoned as sacrosanct contract to share joys of birth of a baby. Though altruistic surrogacy among close relatives where no money changes hands is allowed, the law has in effect completely stopped surrogacy. The experts say the emotional quotient in altruistic surrogacy would make it a non- starter. IVF experts in Delhi, Gujarat and other hubs in different parts of India, practising surrogacy, fumed for they thought the law was mindless one. They implored government to regulate but not banish it altogether.

Ironically, the ban on commercial surrogacy which came as earthquake like shock for the IVF industry shook PM Modi's homeland Gujarat the most. Anand district in Gujarat was not only the seat of Indian milk cooperative but also hub of 'Co-Operative Fertility' wherein an unrelated lady rented her fit womb for birth of child to another childless lady whose womb could not hold embryo.

Surrogacy like Amul is an example of co-operation in fertility. Dr Nayana Patel, a celebrity fertility expert, in Anand, was compared to the Verghese Kurien of co-operative motherhood revolution called Surrogacy. But this veritable baby factory for global clients in Anand has become a thing of the past. The foreigners have completely been barred from availing themselves of this mode of getting children.

The law for banning commercial surrogacy completely, the IVF experts say, is premised on the 'fancy' that surrogate mothers (women mostly poor and downtrodden, who rent their wombs) were exploited and duped. Surprisingly, not even a single such surrogate mother came forward with such complaints of being exploited. Add to it an RTI application asking about such complaints, coming up with answer as none.

On the contrary, lives of poor surrogates got transformed and those who could not make their ends meet were living their lives comfortably in lieu of being an instrument to handing bundles of joy for childless couples. Surrogacy experts complain that the government railroaded the ban without applying its thinking mind. There is no rationale behind clamping it. They said willing surrogate mothers, wanting to better their economic conditions, were even ready to demonstrate in Delhi to call the bluff of baselessly insinuating surrogacy practitioners. The law has allowed only altruistic surrogacy wherein a close relative woman can only provide her womb for child bearing. IVF experts say that altruistic surrogacy is a completely no go, keeping in mind the risk of emotional blackmailing later on.

The experts pulled out all stops to convince powers that be to forestall the passing of the law but no luck. The bill, before becoming law, was open for consultations but the apologists failed to convince the powers that be. Of course, debate raged in the country regarding the merits of the bill but all efforts to save this innocuous practice aborted ultimately. The law has hit multimillion dollar surrogacy biz in one fell swoop to the chagrin of surrogacy advocates. Though there is little hope of revert in foreseeable future and law-abiding IVF centres have called it quits, efforts are still on to get commercial surrogacy restored.

Under the law with strict norms, only proven infertile Indian couples who have been married for at least five years can opt for surrogacy, while those who already have a child cannot do so.

Only Indian nationals are allowed for altruistic surrogacy. Foreign nationals or even NRI or OIC are not to be allowed. Only married couples are allowed to opt of surrogacy. Gay, single, live-in couples are off limits. The marriage should be minimum of five years and the age of the woman should be from 23-50 and for the man 26-55.

The law has penalty provisions for those violating the law, when it comes into effect. The penalties include a huge monetary fine (ten lakh), and imprisonment (ten years) and even striking down the name from medical register. This will increase paper work. The records will have to be kept for five years and not 2 years.

IVF experts roundly called it a humiliation heaped on science. They said a beautiful procedure of splashing around joys among childless couples and in return bringing sunshine to those who were spending their lives in grinding poverty was killed in sheer mindlessness. They just fancied that there must be exploitation galore of poor women renting their womb for money while there was hardly any, evidenced by answer to an RTI application. The answer said not a single evidence of exploiting surrogate mothers was found. They argued that surrogacy should be treated as sacrosanct as society looks at blood donation. If the word commercial rankles, it can be changed with the word compensation. They found themselves at their wits end at seeing this ban being brought without rhyme or reason. They wondered how the government can be so adamant. They alleged the ban was driven by what some NGOs said without checking the facts. The voices of stake holders were not heard. Sane views, respecting regulation, were muffled while making the draft.

Late Sushma Swaraj said while bill was being formulated that she wanted UK surrogacy model to be replicated in India. In UK altruistic surrogacy means that any unknown lady can offer her womb for a compensation of 15,000 pounds. The Indian law allows only free surrogacy. Surrogacy experts said practice of surrogacy in India was also not very different from altruism. There could be no price for having bundle of joys and renting a womb for hapless women longing for motherhood.

In one of the functions on the occasion of opening of a centre just when the bill was being debated, Shilpa Shetty Kundra, the feisty Bollywood Prima Donna, had packed a punch in the last- ditch effort to save commercial surrogacy. Shilpa had powerfully batted in favour of Surrogacy and emphasised the process as an element of women empowerment, the bubbly actor was full throated in her support for Surrogacy and had called it a gift of science. She had said further that womankind should be indebted to science for IVF, test tube baby technique, a great gift as it enables women to procreate. She was unapologetic about the growing trend of having children through renting wombs among denizens of Bollywood. Mrs Shetty had said there was nothing wrong in regulating the process but banishing this process altogether from ART (Assisted Reproductive Technology) was not in the best interest of women.'

Given the world class IVF centres costing very low in comparison to other countries, India was being looked at as 'pregnant' with huge foreign reserve potential, thanks to international commercial surrogacy. Indian wombs could be milch cows for earning foreign revenue for India. This was the plea IVF (Test Tube Baby) lobby was taking in favour of restoration of international surrogacy in India. The issue was raised in MTNL Perfect Health Mela, 2018 in front of the then Ashwini Kumar Choubey, Minister of State for Health and Family Welfare, seeking rethink.

The lobby, which was all for regulation, thinks the moral police has done no good by getting ban clamped on it. Apologists of surrogacy argue how ban has incurred a huge loss of foreign revenue and severed a perennial source of income for poor women including maids, who mostly went for renting wombs. According to them Surrogacy industry of India has gone away to USA, thanks to ban. They say IVF industry has immense potential to bulge India's foreign exchange reserve.

Dr Archana, one of the best IVF experts in the country, at Nurture, says, 'We are all for regulation of surrogacy but banning it has done good to nobody. Surrogacy is a sacrosanct contract to share joys of birth of a baby. Co-Operative Fertility brings joys both to the parents and surrogate mothers.'

Dr Archana Bajaj further says, 'In fact, lives of poor surrogates were being turned around way beyond recognition. One of surrogate mothers for my client became so well off that her daughter now is a doctor. Earlier, she hardly had two meals a day. Ones, who could not make their ends meet, are living their lives comfortably in lieu of being an instrument for handing bundles of joy for childless couples.

She added, 'Surrogacy is a beautiful procedure which splashes joys among childless couples and brings sunshine to those who are living in grinding poverty. It is a win-win situation. Ban on international surrogacy in India, has made USA and Ukraine beneficiary. If allowed, India could become an immense source of revenue generation. We are giving best results in the world in fraction of cost in USA.'

IVF experts still hope good sense might prevail in times to come. They have not fully lost hope. They say it is never too late to mend. But revoking the law banning surrogacy might entail a long-drawn-out labour pain.

Chapter- 12

ART Act: From Trust Raj to Inspector Raj

ART Act is welcome- This was general response from credible practitioners of IVF when it was passed but it seems no more than a cliché and front to sound politically right. It also begets fears of unknown. They fear it might encumber the process. The stated objective of the Act is the regulation and supervision of the assisted reproductive technology clinics and banks.

Though reliable and renowned IVF experts themselves asked for it to salvage their image in the face of allegations flying thick and fast, thanks to unscrupulous fly by night and wannabe operators, the response does not in fact reflect their true outlook about the Act passed by parliament to regulate the domain. Laws in India invariably degenerate and prove the undoing of the very objective it is intended for. ART act and rules therein are not viewed differently. The Act has in actual fact raised the spectre of it proving counterproductive to the industry having potential of making India centre of the universe for having bundles of joy. They would rather have their own internal codes of ethics to regulate them in addition to ICMR guidelines.

The real question behind 'welcome' façade is, will the act really clean practice or be a weapon in the hands of enforcers to harass the good ones in the domain. No doubt there is much rotten in the industry and Augean stable needs to be cleaned. Those who are above board only hope the act does not mess with them. Worries a la inspector raj are staring them. They fear it might inhibit the growth of the fertility industry and create problems instead of solving any. They would have been comfortable practising in trust raj but they acquiesce too in sober fact that it is a wistful thinking, given the unconscionable laissez faire that the industry had degenerated into. Their apprehensions are not ill founded as all laws in India that get passed with stated good intention are taken with a pinch of salt because they are invariably misused. It will be an irony if ART act that has been passed to stop the misuse of IVF, itself becomes the device of misuse.

Indian Society for Assisted Reproduction (ISAR) officials feel the Act needs to be revisited. There are some rough edges which give it a semblance of Draconian, they opine. They fear the law finally might turn out against childless couples and practitioners as well. They say the law which is aimed at preventing misuse, should not be used to create difficulties for persons opting for assisted reproduction methods. Talking to them brings out their reservations about the act. They said while the new Act would streamline practices, certain clauses would discourage small, cost-effective centres, which will turn this legislation into a business model rather than helping highly skilled professional services, especially in smaller towns. Some chapters of ISAR even staged protests to underscore the contentious issues of surrogacy and Assisted Reproductive Technology (ART) Act.

ISAR officials point to report that show India has about 30,000 couples in the reproductive age group suffering from infertility at a given time. The success rate of IVF here is at par with international standards, in spite of the cost being 1/3 of the global fees. As a result, patients come from abroad to seek infertility treatment in India. Only 1 to 2 per cent of the population can avail of services as there still is a lack of awareness with many misconceptions and apprehensions regarding IVF. They claimed it supported the government in bringing out a comprehensive law for ART that can help streamline work, making it more transparent. According to them, the act was the need of the hour but it should not be unfriendly and detrimental to the interest of patients and doctors either.

They said charging of high and recurrent registration fee every five years is highly unjustified and will increase the cost of treatment unnecessarily. Each ART clinic has to pay money to get themselves registered — Rs 5 lakh for five years — with a similar amount required to be paid for surrogacy for the same time period. There is also issue of there being multiple regulating bodies instead of a single one. There must be a single window system of registering and monitoring centres. The offences committed by the doctors during the treatment of surrogacy/ IVF now under the new Act have been made non-bailable and can be punished with five to ten years in prison.

Parliament passed The Assisted Reproductive Technology (Regulation) bill, 2021 that proposed the establishment of a national registry and registration authority for all clinics and medical professionals serving in the field.

Union Health Minister Mansukh Mandaviya while moving the bill for passage in Lok Sabha said several suggestions of Standing Committee have been considered by government to improve the legislation. The bill seeks to regulate and supervise Assisted Reproductive Technology (ART) clinics and ART banks, prevent misuse, adopt safe and ethical practice and so on. Mr Mandaviya had added, 'Many such ART clinics have been running without regulation. A need was felt for regulation of such clinics as there are implications on health of those who undertake the procedure. These bills are aimed to give respect to women facing problems in giving birth.'

Opening the debate, Congress's Karti Chidambaram said this law is Victorian as it does not include lesbian, gay, bisexual or transgender people (LGBTQ) or single men for exercising the right. He also urged the government to consider supporting poor childless parents to take ART's help. Supporting the bill, Dr Heena Gavit of the BJP said the bill sets the minimum standards and codes of conduct for fertility clinics and egg or sperm banks and about 80 percent of ART clinics are not registered. Trinmool Congress (TMC) MP Dr Kakoli Ghosh Dastidar, who is a specialist in the field, said experts should be involved at every level to monitor the Bill's provision and pointed out that ART banks should not be there unless it has proper laboratory, Dastidar and BSP's Sangeeta Azad raised the issue of exclusion of single parents and LGBTQ community from using this procedure. They argued, 'they have a right to be parents too. NCP's Supriya Sule also raised the issue of LGBTQ community and single men being left out. She said, "I think we should not deprive any human being who deserves or wants to have child. Why do we not put right minds together" Ms Sule said that there should not be any jail terms for doctors.

Among other objectives of the Act are ensuring safe and ethical practice of assisted reproductive technology services for addressing the issues of reproductive health where the technology is required for becoming a parent or for freezing gametes, embryos, embryonic tissues for further use due to infertility, and other conditions.

Rules published after passing of Act

The Ministry of Health and Family Welfare on 7th June 2022, has published the Assisted Reproductive Technology (Regulation) Rules, 2022 to regulate the functioning of Assisted Reproductive Technology (ART) clinics and banks.

As per this rule, there shall be two levels of clinics, namely, Level 1 ART Clinics, where only intrauterine insemination (IUI) procedure is carried out as part of treatment and Level 2 ART clinics, where the procedures, or as the case may be, techniques, that attempt to obtain a pregnancy shall be carried out.

The Assisted Reproductive Technology (ART) banks shall-

- Be responsible for screening, collection and registration of the semen donor and cryopreservation of sperms;

- Perform screening and registration of oocyte donor;

- Operate as semen banks or oocyte banks or both;

- Maintain the records or data of all the donors and shall regularly update the National Registry.

An application for registration shall be made by the ART clinics or any such health facility which are carrying out procedures related to assisted reproductive technology, to the appropriate authority in Form-1 and by the ART banks in Form-2.

The appropriate authority shall, after making such enquiry and after satisfying itself that the applicant has complied with all the requirements, shall grant a certificate of registration in Form 3 to the applicant. One copy of the certificate of registration shall be displayed by the registered ART clinic or ART bank at a conspicuous place at its place of business.

Every clinic and every bank shall maintain a grievance cell in respect of matters relating to such clinics and banks and the manner of making a compliant before such grievance cell be as specified in Form 5.

The ART clinic shall ensure that all unused gametes or embryos shall be preserved by the assisted reproductive technology clinic for use on the same recipient and shall not be used for any other couple, or as the case may be, woman and it shall ensure that no pre-implantation genetic testing shall be done for sex selection for non-medical reasons or selection of particular traits due to personal preferences of the prospective parents or to alter or with a view to alter the genetic constitution of an embryo.

Why Regulation was the need of the hour

Shady and fly by night fertility clinics have become rife all over India which are devoid of proper equipment, safety measures and qualified staff resulting even in the death of some patients. Complaints of medical negligence were common. There was unabated mushrooming of such fertility centres which operated with impunity. According to one estimate, a new fertility clinic was being set up every tenth day. Drug overdose, injury to blood vessels, excessive stimulation of the ovaries, water and electrolytes imbalance and kidney failure are some of the major causes of death of Infertility patients. In such substandard clinics danger of death always loomed large.

Questionable and wannabe IVF centres were out to tap into the desperation of childless couples who are increasing by the day. Increasing incidence of infertility prompted them to resort to make a killing by duping them. Hope selling without wherewithal to ensure bundles of joy was rampant. According to one of the surveys done across Indian metros Calcutta, Delhi, Mumbai, Chennai, Kochi, Agra, Bangalore, Hyderabad and Ahmedabad, around 46 per cent of Indian couples aged 31-40 years were found infertile. The crowd at such centres underlined the enormity of infertility. For unscrupulous players, fertility clinics seemed easy money-making propositions. It indeed presented a very lucrative option.

Not surprisingly, the number of IVF clinics is pegged at between 20,000 and 40,000. But registered clinics did not count even 2 thousand. The Indian Council of Medical Research (ICMR) once said there were some 1,200 assisted reproductive technology (ART) clinics in India. Out of which, only 177 are enrolled with the ICMR.

Many of such clinics were found operating in small spaces with outdated equipment. They would have no emergency management systems and utter lack of trained gynaecologists, skilled staff and health assistants. Surprisingly, even such clinics were found brimming with patients. Unsuspecting infertile couples were up for grab by such shady centres.

For a clinic to run professionally, it needs at least one reproductive medicine expert, an embryologist and an andrologist. As regards facilities, in addition to a clean environment, the centre should have a quality incubator which is used for mating eggs and sperm and multiplying embryos. Besides, it should have a storage facility to preserve embryos in frozen conditions. Many of the top clinics meet these requirements.

Chapter- 13

Stem Cells may pack a Punch in IVF

IVF is increasingly advancing with various inventions and innovations amply exemplified by constant jump in success rate in Centres of excellence like Nurture. Stem cell therapy is the latest potential accessory being looked at with much anticipation in IVF domain. The prospect of this value addition on fertility treatment like IVF seems real. Stem Cell Scientists are confident that if stem cell therapy is wedded to IVF, it might boost its success rates still further. For now, this prospect is at best a leap of faith.

Stem cell scientists carry the conviction that the blend of IVF and stem cell therapy will in times to come make take home baby almost a certainty. They claim stem cells possess solutions for all infertility related problems ranging from thin endometrium, low ovarian reserve and ovarian failure in women to low sperm count and azoospermia (complete lack of sperm) in men. Dr (Mrs) Bajaj says, 'Stem cell therapy is yet to come of age in infertility treatment. We are keenly watching how it evolves and come as a value addition on IVF. We would like to see how it pans out and are open to integrate it with our process in Nurture'. Dr Hrishikesh Pai, the Mumbai based ace IVF expert vouches for potential of stem cell therapy in IVF and looks forward to integrating it in his centre.

The introduction of stem cell in IVF treatment is recently developed module which is said to be 'pregnant' with enormous promise. It is believed to be much more effective than the traditional procedure, as it can create undifferentiated cells without any complication. The stem cell therapy is said to quicken the efficiency of the treatment to a great extent. In males, it can cure the issue of sperm production by repairing the tissues. In the females, it can come handy in improving the health of the uterus and making it much more effective. Bone Marrow Aspirate Concentrate (BMAC) is being looked at as game changer in premature ovarian failure.

Prabhu Mishra, an ace stem cell scientist and Medtech entrepreneur holds the brief for effective intervention of stem cell therapy in IVF. As CEO of StemGenn Therapeutics and Founder & President of International Association of Stem Cell and Regenerative Medicine (IASRM), Mr Mishra is optimistic about its major role as an adjuvant to IVF and general treatment of infertility. Prabhu Mishra, who is strong advocate of marriage between IVF and Stem Cells therapy, says, 'Stem cell & Regenerative Medicine especially PRP, BMAC therapies are adjuvant to IVF treatment which acts like bridge between them as it may improve endometrial thickness and follicle quality in ovaries. PRP, BMAC, Adipose stem cells, Ipsc are definitely future of infertility management and need relevant controlled comparative studies for efficacy.'

Globally, regenerative science in infertility treatment presents a robust change in the treatment of premature ovarian failure. In this context, bone marrow aspirate concentrate (BMAC) which contains bone marrow derived mesenchymal stem cells pave a way for better understanding in the biology of ovarian rejuvenation. The scope for further research in bone marrow aspirate concentrate for infertility treatment relies on

a. Standardization of dosage and frequency of the injection,

b. Universal protocol on preparation methods and injection techniques,

c. Immunogenicity of bone marrow aspirate concentrate,

d. Usage of autologous or allogenic preparation,

e. Radiological documentation on ovarian rejuvenation (evidence-based medicine) and

f. Randomized controlled trials to be conducted on BMAC in infertility treatment.

Talking at length about stem cell therapy's seminal role in boosting IVF, Prabhu Mishra further says a relevant amount of data supports the concept that adult stem cells can differentiate either in hematopoietic or non-hematopoietic tissues (1). A large amount of emerging preclinical data drives the introduction of several stem/progenitor cells into regenerative medicine with varied extent of therapeutic benefit. Adult mono nucleated cells, containing the stem cell/ progenitor cell fraction, can be isolated from mobilized peripheral blood and bone marrow tissue using density gradients (2).

Bone marrow has an organized anatomical architecture which facilitates interaction among stem cells amidst a regulatory microenvironment that is composed of endothelial cells, adipocytes, and fibroblasts, along with lymphocytes and macrophages (3, 4). Bone marrow derived stem cells interact with the stroma of the bone marrow through adhesion molecules like very late antigen-4 and cytokine receptors which bind to cytokines that are associated with the membrane/ ligands binding to the extracellular matrix (ECM). Glycoproteins such as G-CSF are shown to interact with the ECM of the bone marrow which decreases the attachment of bone marrow derived stem cells to the stroma thereby promoting their release into the bloodstream (5). The main components of the ECM including collagens, laminins, proteoglycans, and fibronectin play a crucial role in the homeostasis of the bone marrow (6).

Since the first BM transplant was reported (7), autologous and heterologous BM transplantation have been used with success for more than 50 years. Greater experience and further characterization of different BMDSC populations have opened a new translational field for certain incurable degenerative pathologies. The use of BMDSCs as advanced cell therapy is gaining momentum.

BMAC as regenerative medicine for infertility treatment

Tal et al in 2019 provide interesting evidence of mobilization of mouse MSCs from bone marrow to blood circulation during pregnancy (8). They showed that BMSCs circulated to the decidual stroma and differentiated into nonhematopoietic prolactin-expressing decidual cells. Further, nonhematopoietic BMSCs impacted the decidual molecular niche and subsequently improved the implantation. Several other studies confirm that BMSCs can migrate to the endometrium post systemic infusion. Interestingly, bone marrow transplantation between male to female mice model demonstrate that BMSC derived from donor male bone marrow migrates to the uterus of the recipient female mice. The migratory ability of BMSCs was confirmed by the detection of cells expressing SRY gene and Y chromosome in the uterus of female (9). Similarly, in a study donor-derived cells were found in the uterine tissue of a woman who had undergone allogeneic bone marrow transplantation which further confirms BMSC migratory effect (10, 11). These studies indicate that BMSCs may be a promising candidate cells for the reproductive cell replacement.

A number of studies have shown that after injecting BMSCs at the target site, various growth factors were secreted into the endometrium which effectively stimulates microvascular endothelial cell proliferation and differentiation (12, 13). In mouse models, it has been shown that transplantation of BMSCs improves infertility by upregulating markers for endometrial receptivity (14). Zhao et al demonstrate that injecting BMSCs into uterine cavity elevates the expression level of protein marker of endometrial cells thereby resulting in increment of the endometrial thickness of the rat model

(15). This suggests that immunomodulatory and migratory properties of BMSCs enhance endometrial cell regeneration upon infusion. In addition, Wang et al have shown that BMSC transplantation effectively repairs the damage of endometrium, through upregulation of estrogen receptor (ER) and progesterone receptor (PR) levels (16).

According to the first case reported, autologous bone marrow derived stem cells with surface markers CD + 9, CD40+ and CD90+ were placed into the endometrial cavity with the aim to successfully treat AS in a patient undergoing egg donation (17). The second study went on to describe the direct placement of non-characterized mononuclear stem cells into the sub-endometrial zone trough transmyometrial injection however, no reproductive outcomes were evaluated (18). Phase I Clinical Trial with CD133+ bone marrow derived stem cells and vascular endothelial growth factor receptor 2 (VEGFR2) represented the EPC subpopulation (19). EPCs are shown to mobilize to the circulation to improve neo angiogenesis of pre-existing endothelium according to a study and has been used in clinical trials for regenerative medicine in nonhematological applications (20).

Mishra Et Al also suggested.

www.ingramcontent.com/pod-product-compliance
Lightning Source LLC
Chambersburg PA
CBHW062227150726
47991CB00006B/2472